Counselling for Psychosomatic Problems

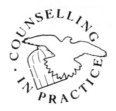

Counselling in Practice

Series editor: Windy Dryden
Associate editor: E. Thomas Dowd

Counselling in Practice is a series of books developed especially for counsellors and students of counselling which provides practical, accessible guidelines for dealing with clients with specific, but very common, problems.

Counselling for Psychosomatic Problems

Diana Sanders

SAGE Publications
London • Thousand Oaks • New Delhi

First published 1996

 SAGE Publications Ltd
6 Bonhill Street
London EC2A 4PU

SAGE Publications Inc
2455 Teller Road
Thousand Oaks, California 91320

SAGE Publications India Pvt Ltd
32, M-Block Market
Greater Kailash – I
New Delhi 110 048

British Library Cataloguing in Publication data

A catalogue record for this book is available from the British
Library.

ISBN 0 8039 7921-5
ISBN 0 8039 7922-3 (pbk)

Library of Congress catalog record available

Typeset by Mayhew Typesetting, Rhayader, Powys
Printed in Great Britain by Biddles Ltd, Guildford, Surrey

Contents

Preface

The effects of psychological factors on our health has been recognized for a long time. In the second century, Galen put forward the idea that the passions, such as anger, lust and fear were important causes of illness. More recently, the field of psychosomatic medicine has looked at psychological causes and correlates of a wide range of physical problems such as asthma, back pain, excema and ulcers, with a growing interest in how stress and our psychological state can influence disease processes. Psychosomatic problems are extremely common. Many of us will notice a range of physical symptoms or problems related to stresses and difficulties in our lives and it is not uncommon for these somatic signs to be used as indicators that our psychological world or lifestyle needs attending to. However, physical problems that appear to be unrelated to obvious or known medical causes can lead to a great deal of distress. The individual may consult a large number of doctors and repeatedly go through medical investigations or treatment, without success, further compounding the problems.

Counselling for Psychosomatic Problems is aimed at counsellors working with people whose physical symptoms are, at least initially, the client's main focus for concern, but where diagnosed organic disease or damage does not account for the symptoms. Instead, psychological factors play a role in causing or maintaining the symptoms. Some of the more common symptoms of concern to this group of clients include chest pains, gastrointestinal problems, headaches, backache, fatigue, pain, unexplained physical sensations such as pins and needles, or breathlessness. Such problems and the accompanying distress may also occur in people with diagnosed physical problems. The book is divided into two parts: Part I is devoted to theoretical issues, Part II to counselling practice.

Part I looks at the background and key issues of working with clients with 'medically unexplained' physical problems. Chapter 1 discusses various definitions and diagnoses of these problems, focusing on the difficulties in clearly defining whether an illness is physical or psychological, given the uncertainties abounding in medicine. It describes some of the psychological categories and terminology used to describe the client group, including hypochondriasis and health anxiety, somatoform disorders and the process of somatization. The chapter discusses the difficulties in language when working with this client group, attempting to get away from definitions and descriptions of the clients' problems as being unreal or all in the mind, and negative connotations of the term psychosomatic. Chapter 2 looks at theories available to account for somatic problems. The main focus of the book is the cognitive behavioural model of the development and maintenance of somatic problems. Chapter 3 addresses key counselling issues in working with clients with psychosomatic problems. The main challenges to counsellors, discussed in this chapter, are to engage the client in counselling and develop a therapeutic relationship in which to work collaboratively with the client, when the client may see their problems as physical, and may therefore be both puzzled and angry at the idea of counselling. The chapter looks at some of the aims of counselling in this area, including helping the client to look at different options as to the cause of their symptoms and to develop effective coping strategies.

In Part II, the process of counselling using a cognitive framework is described in detail, with two case studies as illustrations, leading the reader through the beginning, middle and end of counselling. Chapter 4 looks at the initial stages of counselling and describes how to assess these clients and develop with the client a conceptualization or formulation of the problems and plan for counselling. Chapter 5 offers some of the nuts and bolts of counselling, and practical techniques to help clients to re-evaluate their symptoms and learn practical ways of coping. The importance of working collaboratively with the client, integrating counselling approaches with the individual conceptualization, is stressed. Chapter 6 introduces ideas from schema focused cognitive therapy, looking at how underlying beliefs and themes may maintain the client's problems, and ways of working with these. Obstacles that frequently arise when working with this client group are considered in Chapter 7 and Chapter 8 looks at issues concerned with ending counselling.

As well as covering general issues, the book discusses working with health anxiety and focuses in particular on two specific problems: medically unexplained bowel disorders, including irritable bowel syndrome, and atypical chest pain. These problems have been selected because they are common problems and illustrate many of the key issues in working with clients with psychosomatic problems, and because they are my particular areas of interest and research. However, lest the reader does not share my enthusiasm for bowels and chests, the book also includes information and key references on working with people with other somatic problems.

A note on language

A variety of different terms are used to describe people who present for counselling with somatic problems and the symptoms or problems: people with psychosomatic problems, medically unexplained symptoms, somatization symptoms or functional somatic symptoms. I have used these terms interchangeably throughout the book, except where each term has a specific and idiosyncratic meaning. The terms 'conceptualization' and 'formulation' are used interchangeably in the book. People are described as patients when discussed as users of medical services, such as consulting general practitioners or hospital doctors, otherwise the term client is used.

Acknowledgements

I am very grateful to a number of people in Oxford who have helped me to develop my work in this field, in particular Helen Kennerley, Christopher Bass and Ann Hackmann. Special thanks to Ivana Klimes, who got me started. Jessica Burnett-Stuart, Christine Küchemann, Martina Mueller and Helena Fox have made helpful comments on the manuscript and Susan Worsey at Sage Publications has been supportive and helpful throughout the various stages of the book. Frank Wills has been a much valued source of help, carefully commenting on the manuscript and reminding me of my audience. My partner, Mo Chandler, deserves special thanks for his continual encouragement, help and support, not to mention his reminders to take my eyes off the computer screen. Finally, I am grateful to my clients who, over the years, have taught me a great deal.

PART I: PSYCHOSOMATIC PROBLEMS AND WORKING WITHIN A COGNITIVE FRAMEWORK

1

What are Psychosomatic Problems? Definitions and Diagnoses

Many people regularly experience a range of minor physical symptoms: in fact, some symptoms some of the time seems to be the rule rather than the exception. A large proportion, around 30 to 80 per cent, of people attending general practitioners and medical outpatient clinics have symptoms which cannot be clearly medically diagnosed (Barsky and Klerman, 1983; Creed et al., 1992; Mayou, 1993). Symptoms such as chest or abdominal pains, breathlessness, fatigue, headaches, backaches and gastric problems may not be caused by any serious medical factors or disease, but nevertheless cause a great deal of concern until a medical opinion is obtained. The majority find the symptoms transient and accept that there is nothing seriously wrong; many of these people will think about and discuss their symptoms with friends and family and realize that they have been under stress or worried unnecessarily. A proportion of people, despite a negative physical diagnosis and medical reassurance, continue to believe that something is seriously wrong with them and may seek medical help numerous times, and have numerous tests and investigations, perhaps over many years. They may become extremely anxious about their health and preoccupied with the idea that something is seriously wrong. Eventually, some of these clients may either feel the need for psychological help and support, and seek counselling or may be offered or referred for psychological help by medical practitioners.

As illustrated in Figure 1.1, the pathway to counselling is not straightforward. The individual may have a long history of seeking help, medical investigations or treatment which has not helped their problems and which may have even done some harm. As a result of this journey, the client may be frustrated, distressed, angry and disillusioned with the ability of others to help them. These people have been traditionally poorly managed by the medical profession.

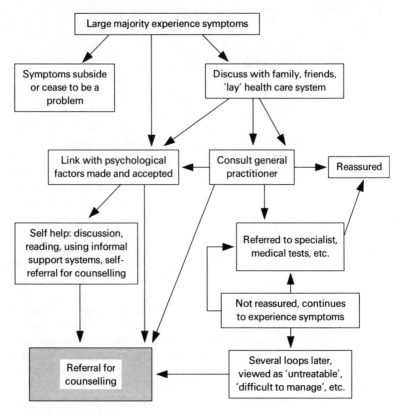

Figure 1.1 *Pathways to referral for psychological therapy for physical symptoms*

They may have had numerous investigations and treatments that have not only used up large amounts of medical resources but also not resolved the problems, and so contributed to further distress and disability (Bass and Benjamin, 1993; Creed et al., 1992; Sharpe et al., 1995). G. Cheyne, writing in 1733, expressed his difficulties and frustrations when trying to help his patients who could not easily be categorized as suffering from known diseases:

> . . . often when I have been consulted in a Case, and found it to be what is commonly called Nervous, I have been in the utmost Difficulty, when desir'd to name the Distemper, for fear of affronting them, or fixing a Reproach on a Family or Person. If I call'd the case 'Glandular with nervous Symptoms', they concluded that I thought them pox'd, or had the King's Evil. If I said it was Vapours, Hysterick or Hypochondriackal Disorders, they thought that I call'd them Mad or Fantastickal; and if

they were such as called themselves, or fearing neither God nor Devil: I was in a Hazard of a Drubbing for seeming to impeach their Courage: and even the very best has been, I myself was thought a Fool, a weak and ignorant Coxcomb, an perhaps dismiss'd in Scorn; and some I have actually lost by it. (Cheyne, 1733, cited in Goldberg et al., 1989)

Unfortunately the difficulties expressed in the eighteenth century still hold true today. People who cannot be easily diagnosed or treated and who repeatedly ask for medical help typically invoke negative reactions, with a whole literature on the 'difficult to manage', 'hard to help', and 'heart-sink patient'. Their distress is frequently dismissed as 'psychosomatic' or 'all in the mind' and therefore unreal, the implication being that the individual has no legitimate cause for complaint. People who frequently attend general practice and hospital clinics with a variety of medically unexplained symptoms have been given various names such as 'crocks', 'turkeys', 'the worried well' and 'the problem patients' (Lipowski, 1988). The negative reactions and tendency to label these people expresses the frustration and problems of those attempting to offer help and does not contribute to a useful understanding of the clients.

A century ago, the puzzle of medically unexplained symptoms led Freud and Breuer to develop concepts such as unconscious conflict, defences and resistance. Freud distinguished between somatic symptoms that were directly caused by excessive nervous activity, the actual neuroses, and those that were indirectly caused by intrapsychic conflict, the neurosis of hysteria. Freud used the term 'conversion' to describe the psychological mechanism whereby nervous energy associated with unexpressed emotion was repressed and transformed into bodily symptoms. Unexplained physical symptoms were considered to be outward signs of psychological disturbances, which became transduced into somatic forms via hysteria and conversion. Patients' insistence that their symptoms were 'real' and 'organic' was taken to represent their defence against the outpouring of intrapsychic conflict (Sulloway, 1979). The idea of the 'transduction' of nervous activity into somatic disease still echoes in psychosomatic medicine, in psychiatric diagnostic categories of somatoform disorders and in modern concepts of somatization. For example, the concept of alexythymia implies that if strong emotions cannot be symbolically transformed and given verbal expression, they are discharged along autonomic pathways, causing psychological disorders (Taylor, 1987).

Definitions of medically unexplained symptoms

There have been many attempts in the psychological literature to categorize and define medically unexplained physical symptoms,

Table 1.1　*Symptoms and syndromes which may be medically unexplained (from Mayou et al., 1995)*

Somatic symptoms	Syndromes
Pain:	
Abdominal	Somatization disorder
Chest	Chronic pain syndromes
Muscle and joint	Irritable bowel syndrome
Low back	Post-traumatic syndromes
Headache	Dysmorphophobia
Facial	Hyperventilation syndrome
Pelvic	Premenstrual syndrome
Neuropathic	Factitious syndromes
Fatigue	Chronic fatigue syndrome
Breathlessness	
Palpitations	
Loss of hearing or ability to speak	
Inability to eat	
Nausea	
Diarrhoea	
Food allergy	
Dizziness	
Incontinence and urgency	
Tremor or shaking	
Worry about benign lumps or skin inconsistencies	
Itching	

both in terms of the physical symptoms themselves and the psychological problems. When considering symptoms that have no clear organic basis, a number of terms have been used, including 'medically unexplained symptoms', 'functional somatic symptoms' and 'somatization symptoms'. The range of medically unexplained symptoms and syndromes is shown in Table 1.1.

It is extremely difficult to define absolutely what constitutes medically unexplained symptoms or syndromes, since the definition assumes that the problems are not caused by physical factors. It is, in fact, almost impossible to say with absolute certainty that an individual does not have, say, heart disease or cancer or some as yet unknown organic cause for their symptoms. A medical diagnosis or opinion is usually one of a degree of certainty rather than an absolute. In addition, medically unexplained symptoms can occur in association with demonstrable physical illness: for example, people with angina caused by diseased coronary arteries may also experience atypical chest pain; irritable bowel syndrome may coexist with inflammatory bowel disease such as diverticulitis or Crohn's disease.

Physical symptoms may also occur where the presence of physical disease is uncertain or disputed, for example, irritable bowel syndrome, premenstrual syndrome and chronic fatigue syndrome (Sharpe et al., 1992). Problems which originally had a physical cause can later be maintained by psychological factors. There is also the possibility that so-called medically unexplained physical symptoms may later turn out to have a measurable organic basis. Many of us know of examples where individuals have been told that their symptoms are not medically serious or are caused by stress, but which later turn out to be caused by explicable organic factors or serious disease. Conversely, as the following illustrates, the individual may have the opposite experience: being told initially that they have a serious physical problem, which later turns out to be benign.

> 'Mary', a 52-year-old school teacher, started to experience several mild attacks of pain in her chest, radiating down her arms, accompanied by feeling breathless, faint and numb in her fingers. The first three times she noticed the symptoms, she rested for a while and the symptoms went away: she attributed them to being tired and overworked by her demanding job and looking after her elderly mother. However, the fourth attack, which happened in the supermarket, was much more severe: Mary collapsed with the pain and the manager called an ambulance. The first doctor to examine Mary said that she had suffered an acute attack of angina and may even have had a heart attack. She stayed in hospital for four days for tests, including an angiogram. She was then told her heart was fine, she did not have angina, and that the pain was 'probably psychosomatic' and to take things easy for a while. Mary continued to experience attacks of pain, and was extremely worried that her symptoms were 'all in her mind' and that she was 'going mad'.

Classifying the psychological distress

Regardless of the relation to organic factors, psychological factors play an important role both in the individual's distress and in the decision to seek help. In practice, the counsellor may well see individuals in the following broad categories:

1 Clients who are suffering from *anxiety* or *depression*, or a combination of both problems. Rather than asking for help for emotional issues, the client will focus on and be concerned about the physical symptoms, at least initially, and may believe that they are physically ill.

2 Clients who are not overtly depressed or anxious, but are experiencing a range of symptoms which cannot be explained by known medical factors. They may be anxious or upset about the symptoms, thereby presenting as suffering from emotional problems. Some of these individuals may be categorized as suffering from *somatoform disorders*.

3 Clients who are both experiencing physical symptoms and are extremely worried and anxious about the possibility of serious medical illness, and who will repeatedly ask for medical opinions, tests or reassurance. These people may be diagnosable as suffering from *health anxiety* or *hypochondriasis*.

These three categories are described in greater detail below.

Depression and anxiety

Physical symptoms characterize many of the psychological disorders (American Psychiatric Association, 1994), and depression and anxiety are well-known causes of many somatic symptoms. An individual who is very low and depressed experiences significant changes in physical functioning, characterized by physical exhaustion, difficulty sleeping or a change in sleeping patterns, loss of appetite or sexual desire, irritability or loss of concentration. The physical experiences may overwhelm or replace the emotions of depression such as loss of enjoyment of life, sadness or hopelessness (Gilbert, 1992). Anxiety is characterized by a wide range of physical symptoms, including chest pains, breathlessness, dizziness, inability to think clearly, faintness, choking, difficulty swallowing, tingling in the hands and feet, sweating or trembling. The experience of a panic attack is overwhelmingly physical, characterized by a combination of intense physical symptoms such as palpitations, pounding heart or accelerated heart rate, sweating, shaking, feelings of choking, chest pains, nausea, dizziness, numbness or hot flushes (American Psychiatric Association, 1994). Not surprisingly, the individual may believe that they are having a heart attack (Clark, 1989; Hallam, 1992). Both depression and anxiety may make the individual more prone to notice physical sensations which may otherwise have been ignored. For example, a headache when rushing through a busy day may not be noticed; but a headache experienced when sitting around feeling low will take on a different significance.

It is frequently these distressing physical symptoms, rather than the underlying emotional problems, that lead the individual to seek help. Around one fifth of new consultations for physical symptoms in primary care are found to be due to primary, or coexisting, anxiety and depression (Bridges and Goldberg, 1985). An emotionally

distressed individual is far more likely to consult a general practitioner with physical symptoms than to consult directly with
emotional or social problems (Murphy, 1989). For example, only 17
per cent of a group of 500 people who met diagnostic criteria for
depression or anxiety directly asked for help with psychological
problems, whereas 56 per cent initially complained of physical
symptoms (Bridges and Goldberg, 1985). Of these people, 24 per cent
readily admitted their psychological problems when asked the right
questions, whereas 32 per cent were what Bridges and Goldberg
called 'pure somatizers', who saw their problems as being entirely
physical and were unwilling to consider psychological factors. This
group were less depressed than the others, and had a less sympathetic
attitude towards mental illness (Bridges et al., 1991). Therefore,
although the individual client may well be depressed or anxious, she
or he may not recognize or want to see that this is the problem. For
these people, part of the initial task for the helper, such as the general
practitioner or counsellor, is to help to identify what the individual's
problems are. Unfortunately, this does not always happen, or may
take time: for example, many people seeking help from the general
practitioner for back pains, headaches or tiredness may receive
numerous physical investigations and treatments before the link is
made with ongoing life problems, stress or depression.

There may be a number of reasons why some psychologically
distressed individuals experience or notice physical symptoms and
worry about these symptoms whereas others focus on their emotional state. Although we all have sensations from the body, we all
differ in our awareness of bodily functions. Research has shown that
individuals who tend to experience physical symptoms rather than
psychological distress are more aware of their bodily functions either
than so-called 'normal' individuals or than those with diagnosable
physical disease. Some individuals seem more ready than others to
ascribe illness explanations to bodily functions, leading to more
distress or anxiety, which can in turn lead to more somatic symptoms. There may be a difference, too, in the relative importance
given to physical symptoms versus psychological distress. Feeling
sad, lonely, down or irritable may be regarded as trivial, and not
worthy of the attention of the medical profession; pain, headaches,
tiredness or palpitations are taken more seriously by both patient
and doctor. Both depression and anxiety may lower the individual's
threshold to pain. Therefore, there is a strong interaction between
physical symptoms and emotional state.

The concept of somatization The term 'somatization' was introduced by Stekel early this century to describe '. . . a deep-seated

neurosis akin to the mental mechanism of conversion' (Bass, 1990). The definition has moved on since then and lost some, but not all, of its psychoanalytic overtones: somatization is generally defined as the process whereby people with psychosocial and emotional distress articulate their problems primarily through physical symptoms (Bass, 1990; Katon et al., 1990; Lipowski, 1988). The concept of somatization requires that the individual both asks for help for a physical complaint and has a diagnosable psychological disorder. In practice, the definition is also used to describe individuals who present with medically unexplained symptoms, but do not have overt psychological problems, rather, having abnormal, unusual or unhelpful health beliefs, such as are found in many people with atypical chest pain and irritable bowel syndrome (Mayou, 1993). Robbins and Kirmayer (1991) distinguish three different types of somatization: somatization as medically unexplained somatic symptoms; somatization as worry akin to hypochondriasis, the tendency to worry about the possibility that one has, or is vulnerable to a serious physical illness; and somatization as the somatic presentation of psychological disorder. The three vary in the extent of somatic symptoms, the extent of anxiety about perceived or actual symptoms, and the extent of psychological disorder.

Somatoform disorders
Although a large number of individuals who initially become concerned about physical symptoms are, in fact, suffering from depression or anxiety, a certain number seem to experience medically unexplained physical symptoms in the absence of significant psychological distress. These people have been a puzzle in attempts to classify and understand their problems. The category 'somatoform disorders' describes 'the presence of physical symptoms that suggest a general medical condition and are not fully explained by a general medical condition, by the direct effects of a substance or by another mental disorder, such as panic disorder' (American Psychiatric Association, 1994). There are eight conditions classified as somatoform disorders in the *Diagnostic and Statistical Manual of Mental Disorders* (American Psychiatric Association, 1994) and *the ICD-10 Classification of Mental and Behavioural Disorders* (World Health Organization, 1993):

- *Undifferentiated somatoform disorder* is characterized by unexplained physical problems lasting at least six months.
- *Conversion disorder* involves unexplained symptoms affecting the individual's motor or sensory functioning that suggest a

neurological or other general medical condition, and where psychological factors are associated with the symptoms.

- *Somatoform pain disorder* is characterized by pain being the main problem, with psychological factors involved in causing, maintaining or exacerbating the pain.
- *Somatoform autonomic dysfunction*, characterized by symptoms of autonomic nervous system activity – such as palpitations, sweating, chest pains, increased bowel activity or need to urinate, or tiredness – which the individual attributes to physical disorder whereas there is no objective evidence of physical disease or disorder.
- *Hypochondriasis* is the preoccupation with the fear of having, or the belief that one has, a serious disease, based on the individual misinterpreting his or her physical symptoms or functions.
- *Body dysmorphic disorder* is the preoccupation with an imagined or exaggerated defect in physical appearance.
- *Somatoform disorder not otherwise specified* includes problems characterized by unexplained physical symptoms not meeting the above criteria.
- *Somatization disorder*, historically referred to as hysteria or Briquet's syndrome, is defined as a combination of physical problems including pain, gastrointestinal, cardiovascular, genitourinary, sexual and neurological symptoms, beginning before the age of 30 and extending over a period of years. These individuals may have a long history of unexplained physical symptoms, often starting in childhood, with a long history of repeated medical consultations and referral to many medical specialities for investigations that repeatedly prove negative. Despite negative tests, the individual, and often their family, firmly believe that there is something wrong: the problem is not so much fear of serious illness, characterizing hypochondriasis, but both conviction in disease and repeated medical attendance. These individuals are the least likely to think that counselling or any psychological approach is relevant to them.

These criteria and classifications tend, in practice, to be used more in psychiatric circles than among counsellors. However, it is useful to be aware of the types of classification that are used, and also their limitations. Overall, the classification of somatoform disorders contains four key points of value to understanding the individual's problems:

- The individual is experiencing a range of physical symptoms or problems.
- While some of these symptoms may mimic serious disease, to the

best of medical knowledge, the individual is not likely to be suffering from serious disease.
- Despite this, the individual believes that physical factors entirely or almost entirely explain the symptoms.
- It is likely that a wide range of psychological factors are involved in causing, maintaining or exacerbating the symptoms.

A vast number of people experience medically unexplained physical symptoms: for example, around 15 to 20 per cent of people in Western countries may suffer from irritable bowel syndrome at some time in their lives, and atypical chest pain is found in up to a half of patients in cardiac and emergency clinics. In contrast, somatoform disorders are rare and qualitatively and quantitatively different. On first inspection, the behaviour of an individual who may meet the criteria for a somatoform disorder appears normal: they have a physical complaint and consult the doctor for tests, treatment, certificates and reassurance. Most of us have, at some time, consulted a doctor in a panic about a symptom which turned out to be benign or harmless. Looked at longitudinally, however, the individual may have a lifetime of physical complaints and frequent use of medical resources when not medically indicated, suggesting that there are problems in both the individual and the management by the medical profession. The person may consult about and discuss their physical problems frequently, using not only the conventional medical system as a source of reassurance and advice, but also their friends and family, the media and complementary practitioners. The opinions of others and results of even the most invasive tests and operations may make little difference to the symptoms or behaviour. The problems are often apparent by adolescence and accompanied by personal and social problems throughout life (Bass and Murphy, 1995). The following example illustrates some of the issues in an individual with a long history of unexplained physical problems.

'Lesley', aged 30, is an only child who lives with her mother. She has suffered from repeated aches and pains throughout her childhood, necessitating weeks off school and frequent visits to the doctor. Despite numerous tests, no physical abnormalities can be found to account for her symptoms. Lesley left school at 16 and worked for four years. She did not enjoy her job and her symptoms began to get worse. She left her job, and has not worked since then. She experiences daily attacks of pain and sickness, which she responds to by going to bed. She is not anxious or worried about the symptoms, but consults her doctor every week to ask for further referrals and tests. She stays at home with her mother who looks after her, and who also has a history of chronic, unexplainable back pains and other physical symptoms. She is now doing a training in dressmaking, a job which she feels will accommodate her disability and allow her frequent time off work.

Hypochondriasis or health anxiety
The term hypochondriasis refers to a subgroup of somatoform disorders where the individual is extremely anxious about the possibility of serious illness. The American Psychiatric Association (1994) defines two main components. First, the individual is preoccupied with the fear of having, or the belief that she or he has, a serious disease. Second, the fear of having, or belief that one has, a disease persists despite medical reassurance. Appropriate physical evaluation does not support the diagnosis of any physical disorder that can account for the physical symptoms, and the symptoms are not just symptoms of panic attacks. The beliefs about the symptoms may arise from the individual misinterpreting a range of physical sensations as evidence of disease (Salkovskis, 1989).

Hypochondriasis or health anxiety may coexist with physical symptoms or changes in bodily functions. For example, an individual with irritable bowel syndrome may have measurable and observable changes in bowel function. If also extremely concerned about the possibility that the symptoms indicate bowel cancer which no one has yet diagnosed and the anxiety persists despite medical reassurance, the individual may have both irritable bowel syndrome and hypochondriasis. Another individual may be extremely concerned about the possibility of bowel cancer, and continues to believe in the possibility of bowel cancer in the absence of any functional bowel changes and repeated negative investigations: in this case, the person may have diagnosable hypochondriasis but not irritable bowel syndrome. However, repeated checking, repeated visits to the toilet, straining when emptying bowels, fear of incontinence, not to mention frequent invasive medical tests, may cause changes in how the bowel functions and so lead to irritable bowel syndrome.

Life events and somatic problems

A large amount of research shows that the experience of threatening life events, particularly those involving the loss or threatened loss of close emotional bonds, can lead to both physical and emotional problems. Threatening life events such as bereavement may also precede medically unexplained physical problems (Craig, 1989). The symptoms they experience may resemble those experienced during the terminal illness of the person who died, as the following example illustrates.

'Teresa' had been extremely troubled with attacks of severe and stabbing lower abdominal pain for six years. The pains woke her during the night and she frequently cried out or screamed with pain. No physical problem had been identified despite numerous tests and stays in hospital. During the assessment for counselling, she talked about the death of her mother from ovarian cancer. She wept as she vividly described her mother's uncontrollable pain and eventual death. She rubbed her abdomen as she spoke. 'My pains are just like my Mum's: the same place: and she died.'

It is also possible that the response to stressful life events is determined by the nature of the stress and how acceptable it is to be upset. For example, distress following a death may be acceptable and the individual is expected to be very upset, mourn, expect the support of others and take time off usual activities. However, a similar upset following the break up of a significant relationship, a termination of pregnancy or miscarriage, or transfer at work causing the loss of important working relationships or loss of status and role, may not be culturally acceptable causes of emotional distress and may not lead automatically to additional social support from others. Therefore, an individual may seek help for counselling following a bereavement but may ask the general practitioner for pain killers or a referral to a cardiologist following redundancy.

Issues for counselling for psychosomatic problems

The concepts and categories of medically unexplained symptoms, somatoform disorder, hypochondriasis and somatization pose a dilemma for clients and for those attempting to help them. When hearing the clients' stories, we are always aware of the possibility that their symptoms are indeed caused by physical disease or damage, in which case their concern and consultation behaviours may well be justified and helpful. However, if their symptoms are indeed not as serious or threatening as the client fears, then their response may well be unhelpful and motivated by psychological issues. This leads to uncertainly in both client and counsellor about when it is appropriate to offer psychological help and when to support the client in the search for a medical answer.

Unlike many of the clients making up a counsellor's case load who come for help with psychological problems, relationship difficulties or when faced with difficulties in life, the group of clients with unexplained physical symptoms may both be reluctant to see any psychological therapist and be difficult to engage in counselling. They may not see the relevance of counselling to their problems, or see it as a last resort. Frequently, as illustrated in Figure 1.1, the clients have a long history of medical investigations or treatment, and may have had confusing information about their problems, further compounding their distress and difficulties. It is more usual for these clients to be referred from other sources, such as general practitioners or medical specialists, than it is for them to refer themselves for counselling. This presents particular challenges for the counselling relationship, in the way in which the client engages in counselling and the way in which client and counsellor conceptualize the client's problems. Ways of understanding and conceptualizing psychosomatic problems are discussed in the next chapter.

2

Understanding Psychosomatic Problems

It is only comparatively recently that attention has been paid to ways of effectively helping people with psychosomatic problems. As discussed in the previous chapter, these people have tended to be dismissed as 'hypochondriacs' or 'difficult to manage', or have been referred and assessed throughout the medical system without a full understanding of what, exactly, the individual's problems are. Despite there being clear psychological factors involved in the problems, not many have been offered psychological therapies or counselling.

However, there has been growing interest in the last decade or so in ways of helping these people. Much of the research and development of new psychological therapies has arisen within cognitive therapy. For this reason, the cognitive model and cognitive therapy is given most attention in this book. However, other forms of therapy have added a great deal to understanding this group of clients (Bass, 1990; Kirmayer and Robbins, 1991). These include brief dynamic psychotherapy (Guthrie, 1995; Guthrie et al., 1991, 1992, 1993); group psychotherapy (Melson et al., 1982); techniques of reattribution (Gask et al., 1989; Goldberg et al., 1989); problem solving therapy (Wilkinson and Mynors-Wallis, 1994); and behaviour therapy (Warwick and Marks, 1988). Family therapy may be valuable; systemic approaches may be particularly helpful where it is felt that the symptoms play a useful role within the family structure, such as preventing a spouse leaving the relationship or where the family's illness model maintains one member in the sick role (Watson, 1985).

Cognitive therapy and psychosomatic problems

Cognitive therapy originated some 30 years ago in America as an effective therapy for depression, anxiety and other psychological problems (Beck, 1976; Beck et al., 1979, 1985). More recently cognitive therapy has been adapted for helping people whose main concern is with physical problems or symptoms, either in the presence or absence of organic disease. For example, cognitive approaches are increasingly being used in pain management (Philips, 1987), in rehabilitation following myocardial infarction, and to help people adjust to long-term or terminal illnesses. There is increasing work on the applications and adaptations of cognitive therapy to the area of somatic problems which are not primarily caused by or the result of physical disease, and which may or may not coexist with psychological disorders. Much of the work has arisen from cognitive models of panic disorder (Clark, 1986) and hypochondriasis (Warwick and Salkovskis, 1989, 1990).

The cognitive model links the client's individual vulnerabilities, core beliefs about themselves and their susceptibility to illness, with physical and psychological symptoms and their maintenance. It looks at how the individual interprets or misinterprets physical symptoms as evidence that they have serious medical problems, leading to a vicious circle of worrying about the symptoms, further symptoms and further emotional distress. The cognitive model includes three aspects:

1 A link between thoughts, behaviours, emotions and physical factors, which interact in a vicious circle to *maintain* the problem. Cognitive therapy has, in particular, focused on patterns of thinking and the way thoughts influence our feelings.
2 Triggers and critical incidents that *precipitate* the problem.
3 Unhelpful attitudes and beliefs that *predispose* the individual to developing the problem.

A fourth aspect, particularly important when looking at somatic problems, is the wider social context which may influence all three levels: cultural norms and expectations, the medical profession and tendency to diagnose psychological problems by exclusion rather than make positive diagnoses, and familial and other social factors.

The maintenance of physical symptoms

Central to the cognitive model of the maintenance of physical symptoms is the way the individual thinks about and interprets symptoms. If she or he notices physical sensations and interprets these as symptoms of disease, the client is likely to feel emotionally upset or distressed, behave in a certain way which exacerbates the symptoms and seek medical or other reassurance, which may in turn cause further anxiety and further symptoms.

Body sensations
Bodily sensations can arise from many sources, including innocent physiological changes, such as those experienced during the menstrual cycle, during exercise or when tired, or simply for 'no apparent reason'; sensations and symptoms arising from low mood,

depression or anxiety, and symptoms of minor or major physical disease or damage. How aware we are of such sensations varies between individuals: for example, people vary in the extent they notice tiredness, discomfort or pain. Although external factors, such as lack of stimulation, may increase the individual's focus on symptoms (Pennebaker and Watson, 1991), people vary in the amount they attend to or focus on bodily sensations depending on the meaning given to the sensations. If we believe certain sensations or symptoms are dangerous, we are more likely to pay attention to them and to ignore information or sensory input which does not fit with our beliefs (Barsky et al., 1988). For example, people with irritable bowel symptoms who seek medical help are significantly more likely to pay attention to physical factors and minimize or ignore psychological and stress-related factors in their lives, in comparison to a group of people with IBS symptoms who did not seek medical help (Drossman et al., 1988).

Cognitions
A more crucial aspect is not the sensations themselves but the accompanying thoughts and the meaning the individual attributes to the sensations. Salkovskis and Warwick have stressed the importance of the misinterpretation of bodily changes or symptoms and information about health in leading to and maintaining anxiety about health issues. For example, an attack of chest pain may lead the person to think 'I'm having a heart attack'; changes in bowel habits may be accompanied by thoughts of bowel cancer; a headache may lead to thoughts or images of brain tumours. As well as thoughts about illness, the individual may believe that the consequences of the illness would be particularly catastrophic (Salkovskis, 1989). Bodily functions then become a focus of attention, and the individual may notice previously undetected bodily sensations. These are in turn interpreted as signs of pathology, and may lead to actual changes in physical functioning. Paying attention to pain, for example, increases the experience of pain (Melzack and Wall, 1988). The thoughts and beliefs about the symptoms may arise from observing and falsely interpreting a range of bodily signs and sensations, information from the media, misunderstanding information from medical practitioners, or from unclear or incorrect information from medical practitioners (Salkovskis, 1989).

Emotional response
Taking the symptoms as evidence of disease will lead, understandably, to anxiety, concern or upset. Emotional distress and arousal is, in turn, accompanied by bodily sensations, such as

Table 2.1 *Links between symptoms, thoughts and feelings*

Symptoms	Thoughts	Emotion	Possible mechanisms
Chest pain	Heart attack	Anxiety	Chest wall pain, oesophagitis, hyperventilation, panic attack
Palpitations	Heart attack	Anxiety	Excessive awareness of cardiac rhythm
Breathlessness	Stop breathing, suffocate	Anxiety	Hyperventilation, panic attack, etc.
Abdominal pain, bowel function	Bowel cancer, incontinence	Anxiety, embarrassment	Sympathetic activity
Fatigue	Cannot perform	Depression	Inactivity, depression, over-stressed
Dizziness, faintness	Collapse	Panic	Hyperventilation
Headache	Stroke, tumour	Anxiety	Tension
Chronic pain	Damage, disability, unable to cope	Depression, fear	Various

Source: from Mayou et al. (eds) 1995. *The Treatment of Functional Somatic Symptoms* (Table 7.1). By permission of Oxford University Press.

palpitations, pain from muscular tension, headaches, sweating and so on; low mood may lead to fatigue, muscular pain and a lowered threshold to pain. The individual then notices and pays attention to the symptoms, interprets them as further evidence of illness, and becomes more concerned or upset. The emotional response may also influence the individual's need to seek help: for example, the decision to consult the general practitioner for irritable bowel syndrome is affected by how depressed or anxious the patient feels, independent of symptom severity.

Some common symptoms, associated thoughts and emotions, and postulated mechanisms, are summarized in Table 2.1.

Behaviours
As a result of concern about the symptoms, the individual develops ways of coping with them which may exacerbate the symptoms and so maintain the problem. Behaviours include rubbing or scratching a skin rash, poking a sore area, repeatedly swallowing, over-breathing in response to chest pain, taking medication, reading medical literature, lying down or resting when experiencing fatigue or chest pains. The client may start doing things in the belief that they are

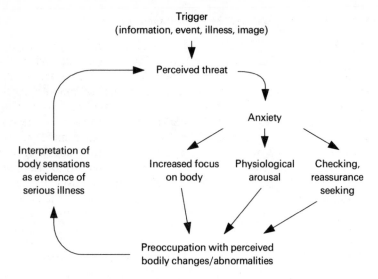

Figure 2.1   *Factors maintaining physical symptoms and anxiety about health*

Source: from Hawton et al. (eds), 1989. *Cognitive Behaviour Therapy for Psychiatric Problems* (Figure 7.1). By permission of Oxford University Press.

preventing a catastrophe from happening. Such 'safety behaviours' include stopping activities when experiencing chest pain, which is thought to avert a heart attack, or wearing nappies when going out in case of incontinence (Salkovskis, 1991; Spoto and Williams, 1987). The person may reduce the normal level of activity, such as taking time off work or avoiding walking or lifting. Although, in the short term, this may relieve the symptoms, there may be long-term detrimental effects. If the individual rests excessively, this may lead to muscle wastage, leading in turn to greater pain or fatigue on exertion, which is then interpreted as a sign of illness. Resting may increase the time the individual has available to notice or pay attention to symptoms. Discussing the symptoms with others may serve to intensify rather than reduce concern. Alternatively, the individual may increase the level of activity, over-doing activities as a means of keeping going, or in response to a time when not feeling so well. Too much activity may exacerbate some symptoms, such as pain or fatigue.

These four aspects – the symptoms, thoughts, emotional response and behaviours – interact to form a vicious circle, as illustrated in Figure 2.1.

Iatrogenesis and psychosomatic problems

As well as the client's behaviour, it is also useful to look at the behaviour of the medical profession in the development and maintenance of psychosomatic problems. Once an individual consults with physical symptoms, the usual course is for the general practitioner to attempt to diagnose or eliminate organic disease before, or as well as, considering psychosocial factors (Porter and Gorman, 1989). Obviously, this is entirely appropriate medical care most of the time; the problem arises when tests repeatedly prove negative, and the individual is repeatedly sent for further investigations to 'rule out' organic disease. Doctors who are interested in psychiatry and psychological factors are more likely to make a positive diagnosis of psychological problems and offer the patient appropriate psychological help than are those who 'diagnose by exclusion', and offer consultations and tests to exclude physical disease before considering psychological factors (Gask et al., 1989; Goldberg et al., 1989, 1992). The range of tests offered in the attempt to exclude organic disease may include barium meal, sigmoidoscopy, venography, mammography, laparoscopy, angiography, EEGs, ECGs, EMGs, X rays, CT scans, MRI scans, endoscopy, ultrasound, lumbar punctures, as well as surgery such as hysterectomy, tonsillectomy and cholecystectomy. There are several reasons why 'frequent attenders' are repeatedly investigated, including the doctor having doubts that organic disease has remained undetected in previous investigations or being unconfident about making an alternative, non-organic diagnosis, or the patient and/or relatives requesting or demanding further tests (Creed et al., 1992). There is little doubt that such investigations can increase the client's belief that there is something wrong (Craig and Boardman, 1990). Further, investigations themselves carry a risk of morbidity and mortality as the following example illustrates.

> 'Dan' had experienced abdominal pains for many years. After a lifetime of consultations and investigations, his gall bladder was removed, an operation which was later thought to be medically unnecessary. The surgery was not successful and led to internal scarring and consequent pain, which severely exacerbated both his somatic symptoms and psychological distress.

Once tests prove negative, the patient is offered reassurance that the symptoms are not caused by serious medical disease; while well meant, reassurance may in itself contribute to the maintenance of physical problems and associated anxiety. It may be phrased in a way that is far from reassuring, such as 'there is nothing sinister found on the tests, but if the symptoms persist, come back and we'll refer you to the hospital for further tests' or 'your blood pressure is not bad for someone of your age' (Salkovskis and Warwick, 1986; Warwick and Salkovskis, 1985). To many, this kind of message is fine, and the individual is reassured. However, for certain people, the message may intensify the anxiety. Medical reassurance may not address the individual's concerns: being told there is 'nothing wrong' is incorrect because the individual is experiencing real symptoms or problems. The medical advice may be ambiguous, such as 'take it easy' or 'don't worry'. Alternatively, doctors may give a diagnosis and offer treatment which later turns out to be incorrect. The following illustrates an example where the medical reaction to symptoms led the individual both to fear the symptoms, and to disbelieve medical opinion.

'Bill' was referred for counselling with abdominal pain, with no apparent cause. The pain was usually worse at night. A few years previously he had been admitted to hospital after a severe bout of pain and was told that it might be rectal cancer. Following an operation to investigate, he was told that he did not have cancer after all, but the pain was caused by a 'spasm in the bowel'. When the symptoms persisted, he was then told it was 'stress' but found this hard to believe: 'How can I be stressed when I'm asleep at night?' His previous experience also led to reluctance to accept theories about 'stress'. Eleven years earlier, he had started to experience attacks of giddiness and stiffness on wakening. He was referred to a psychiatrist, who initially put his problems down to the effects of his difficult childhood. Luckily, the psychiatrist was not convinced this was the whole story and referred Bill to a neurologist, who diagnosed Parkinson's disease. Not surprisingly, Bill is now suspicious of any simplistic psychological explanations of his physical symptoms.

To summarize, the maintenance of physical symptoms depends on an interaction between symptoms and sensations, focusing on and paying attention to the symptoms, interpretation of the meaning of the symptoms, and behaviours including seeking medical reassurance or investigations. The medical system may also influence the maintenance, as well as development, of psychosomatic problems.

To illustrate the points made above, the next section looks at irritable bowel syndrome and atypical chest pain. These problems have been chosen since they are relatively common among individuals seeking counselling and may well be experienced as part of other problems such as anxiety or panic attacks.

Irritable bowel syndrome and atypical chest pain

Irritable bowel syndrome (IBS) is defined as persistent abdominal distension, discomfort or pain, generally relieved by defecation, and an alteration in bowel habits such as alternating diarrhoea and constipation, sometimes accompanied by passage of mucus and a sensation of incomplete evacuation (Farthing, 1995; Stevens and Jones, 1993). Other symptoms include nausea and vomiting, and excessive wind; women sufferers of IBS have an increased incidence of dyspareunia or pain during sexual intercourse. Many people with IBS have a history of abdominal pain from childhood.

Around 17 to 20 per cent of the general population suffer from IBS; however, only a small proportion of people with IBS seek medical advice for their symptoms (Kettell et al., 1992; Stevens and Jones, 1993). Three factors are important in determining medical consultation: severity of symptoms, anxiety about the symptoms and degree of psychological distress (Kettell et al., 1992; Lydeard and Jones, 1989). Recent life difficulties may lead an individual to seek help for irritable bowel symptoms (Creed, 1995; Toner et al., 1990a). In a large number of cases, dietary factors are involved, and elimination diets to exclude possible food allergies or intolerance may be effective, but for some individuals dietary factors do not appear to be so relevant. Other factors thought to be involved in IBS include increased sensitivity to pain. The pain of IBS can be reproduced when a balloon inserted into the colon is inflated, and people with IBS are particularly sensitive to this pain, developing it at a lower volume of balloon distension than those without IBS (Swarbrick et al., 1980). These characteristics of IBS suggests that understanding the problem needs to include an assessment of the role of anxiety and depression and stressful events in precipitating and maintaining symptoms, and the role of individual beliefs and assumptions regarding health. Further questions relate to why the individual made the decision to consult for medical help and why at that particular time.

Irritable bowel syndrome can be extremely disabling for the individual. Some clients may be severely restricted in their activities and may have some degree of agoraphobia. The restrictions often arise from the fear of incontinence or of embarrassing or socially unacceptable symptoms such as wind. Some may have been incontinent as a result of the bowel symptoms, and may have developed a range of ways of coping with the situation, such as avoiding social situations, using laxatives or anti-diarrhoea medication, straining when emptying the bowel, or clenching up abdominal or bowel muscles, which increases the individual's focus on symptoms and may alter bowel function.

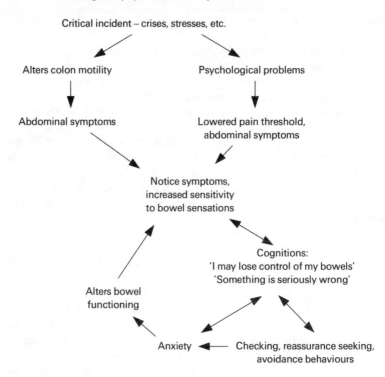

Figure 2.2   *A model of irritable bowel syndrome (from Salkovskis, 1992a; Creed et al., 1992)*

A possible model for IBS is illustrated in Figure 2.2. The model proposes that difficult life events may lead to bowel symptoms either directly, with stress affecting gut motility (Thompson et al., 1992), or indirectly through the development of anxiety or depression. The effects of anxiety on the gut are well established in our language, with terms such as 'scared shitless', 'a gut reaction', 'sickening' and 'gut-wrenching', and describing something or someone as a 'real bellyache'. The resulting symptoms are noticed, leading to thoughts about serious illness, cancer, or lack of control over bowel function, causing further anxiety. The ways the individual develops to cope with the symptoms may be forms of 'safety behaviours' similar to those used by people with agoraphobia or panic attacks, such as only going out where the individual knows the availability of toilets, or escaping from situations when they notice abdominal fullness, inferring that had they not escaped they might have been incontinent (Salkovskis, 1989). Although safety behaviours may reduce the client's anxiety in the short term, in the long term they can lead to further anxiety and also prevent the individual from learning that what they fear is not likely to happen.

Atypical chest pain is thought to affect between 7 and 16 per cent of the general population. Around half of people who are referred to cardiac clinics are found not to have heart disease or other serious physical problem and 20 per cent of cardiac catheterizations are normal, representing 12,000 cases in the UK each year. Of those who are found to have normal coronary arteries, the majority have a normal expectation of life and a normal physical prognosis; however, between 50 and 70 per cent continue to experience symptoms, worry about heart disease, restrict their activities and seek medical help (Bass et al., 1983; Lantinga et al., 1988; Mayou, 1989). People with a variety of psychological problems, including anxiety and hypochondriasis, suffer from chest pain and are worried about heart disease (Potts and Bass, 1994; Salkovskis, 1992b). Around half of people with chest pain and normal coronary arteries are also suffering from psychological problems, mainly anxiety or depression. Conversely, around half of people with atypical chest pain have no obvious psychological problems, but it is possible that their concern about the symptoms and limitation of activity, as well as medical investigations or treatments, may lead to psychological distress. Atypical chest pain can also coexist with coronary disease and angina. A cognitive model of atypical chest pain is shown in Figure 2.3.

The symptoms of pain are thought to arise from a variety of cardiac and non-cardiac sources including micro vascular coronary artery disease, Prinzmetal's angina, or coronary spasm, chest wall pain, oesophageal dysmotility or reflux, or hyperventilation (Potts and Bass, 1994; Salkovskis, 1992b). Whatever the cause of the symptoms, how the individual responds to the symptoms depends on the interpretation. The most common, understandable and, in some cases, most useful reaction is to interpret the sensations as evidence of an impending heart attack. This interpretation is based on a number of factors. Given the high rates of heart disease in the population and the attention given to the subject in the media, notably the explosion of television programmes focusing on the emergency services, most people equate chest pain with a heart attack and its consequences. A number of clients may have had direct experience of heart disease, such as illness or death among relatives, friends or work colleagues, and some may have witnessed a friend or relative having a myocardial infarction. Although many of the general population have lost friends or relatives from heart disease, individuals with atypical chest pain may have had more –

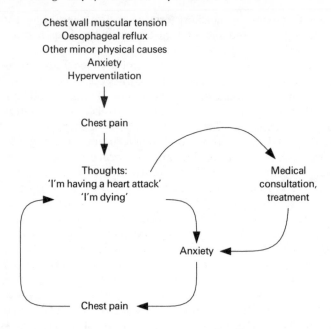

Figure 2.3   *A model of atypical chest pain (Salkovskis, 1992b; Pearce et al., 1990)*

and more upsetting – experiences. People under the age of 40 who present in casualty departments with acute, non-cardiac chest pain have experienced significantly more stressful life events, including bereavements, during the previous year than matched controls (Roll and Theorell, 1987), and Burns and Nichols (1972) found that a group of depressed patients with chest pain reported more recent bereavements, including witnessing a death, compared to a group of depressed patients without chest pain. Interpreting the symptoms as signs of an impending heart attack may also be the most useful interpretation: if it was the case that the individual was indeed having a heart attack, they would be more likely to seek help.

The interpretation of the symptoms leads, not surprisingly, to fear and anxiety, which then exacerbates the chest pain in three ways:

- The individual experiences autonomic arousal, leading to increased heart rate, increased muscular tension, and other symptoms which target the chest area and may exacerbate the chest pain. Terms such as 'broken hearted' may describe the somatic sensations accompanying grief.

- The individual may over breathe or hyperventilate, which may directly cause further chest pain or lead to a range of physical symptoms, such as giddiness and palpitations, that may be interpreted as evidence of a heart attack. Around half of individuals with chest pain can reproduce the symptoms by hyperventilating (Bass et al., 1991).
- The individual attempts to control the symptoms and decrease the likelihood of a heart attack by controlling the breathing, such as breathing in a shallow way while the lungs are expanded, which in turn exacerbates the symptoms.

The first response, sometimes initiated by others, is to seek medical help, often as a medical emergency. The individual may have a range of medical investigations, sometimes including coronary angiography, to exclude or make a positive diagnosis of heart disease. This may lead to a definite conclusion that the person does not have heart disease, discussion about the role of anxiety and panic in chest pain, and the individual may go home reassured. However, in many cases, the person will be given contradictory information, or even a positive diagnosis of angina; they may be prescribed a range of cardiac medication, which is often continued in people with chest pain despite normal coronary arteries, leading to conflicting signals for the individual. Others may be told, definitively, that they do not have heart disease, but are not given a satisfactory explanation of what *is* causing the symptoms. Some emerge from hospital after numerous frightening and painful cardiac investigations with only a 'negative' diagnosis; not surprisingly, the information is difficult to believe.

An important question in understanding the maintenance of chest pain is why the individual continues to experience anxiety and believe that their symptoms are dangerous even after perhaps years of suffering attacks of chest pain but never having had a heart attack. One reason may be that they disbelieve medical information, due to personal experience of medical mismanagement or misdiagnosis. They may believe, perhaps correctly, that if they do not have heart disease now, they will do some time in the future, due to having several risk factors or a family history of heart disease. As for panic disorder, people with chest pain also engage in a number of 'safety behaviours' to prevent the possibility of a heart attack: sitting down, resting or slowing down when experiencing chest pain. While these actions may relieve the symptoms, they also prevent the individual from learning that the chest pains are not linked to an impending heart attack: she or he may continue to believe 'If I had not sat down when I got the pain, I may have had a heart attack', because the effects of carrying on despite the pain have never been tested out (Salkovskis, 1991, 1992b).

Assumptions and beliefs underlying psychosomatic problems

The second aspect of the cognitive model proposes that our individual assumptions and beliefs about ourselves, others and the world underlie how we react to situations and circumstances, and may make us vulnerable to certain problems (Persons, 1989). We all have a set of assumptions and beliefs, or 'frames of reference', which we have learned from relationships with parents, siblings and peers and from our experiences, particularly during childhood. Because of the developmental stage at which we learn these attitudes and beliefs, they become incorporated into our very way of seeing ourselves, others and the world, and may therefore remain unchallenged. Some of our attitudes and beliefs may be helpful and sufficiently flexible to allow us to adapt to changes in ourselves and our worlds. However, if the assumptions are held as unconditional and unhelpful rules, we are more likely to be vulnerable to difficulties. The cognitive model distinguishes between our *assumptions* or *attitudes*, which form our rules for living, and core beliefs or *schema*, relating to basic and central ways of understanding ourselves and the world. Assumptions may relate to the way we function in the world, such as 'In order to be happy, I must be loved by others' or 'I must be successful and never make mistakes', whereas schema reflect unconditional, core beliefs, such as 'I am a bad person' or 'I am vulnerable'. Beck et al. (1990) and Young (1990) discuss assumptions and schema in greater detail.

The kinds of assumptions and beliefs underlying psychosomatic problems can be divided into two main areas: first, those concerning the meaning of physical symptoms, influencing the extent to which the individual sees him or herself as vulnerable to serious illness and its consequences; and second, beliefs concerning the meaning of psychological distress, which influence the way in which the person deals with difficulties and stresses. These two areas are described below, with some ideas about early experiences which may have led the individual to develop their idiosyncratic assumptions and beliefs.

*Assumptions and beliefs about the meaning of physical
symptoms: themes of vulnerability and danger*
There are two areas where beliefs may influence concern about health or health anxiety: beliefs about the meaning of physical symptoms and beliefs about the self, viewing the self as vulnerable

to illness. Certain assumptions may lead the individual to interpret physical symptoms or perceived physical changes as dangerous (Warwick and Salkovskis, 1989, 1990). These may include: 'my body should always function perfectly; any symptoms must indicate something is seriously wrong'; 'if I get an illness, it will be untreatable'; 'both sides of the body must be identical or there is something wrong'; 'symptoms inside the body are more serious than those on the outside'; 'symptoms always mean something serious or they would not be there'; and 'if you don't go to the doctor as soon as you notice anything unusual it may be too late'. People with hypochondriasis may have specific beliefs about health professionals, such as 'if I have symptoms, the doctors should be able to explain and treat these symptoms'. Alternatively, the person may perceive health professionals as likely to make potentially fatal errors of diagnosis, based on personal experience or because of examples from the media (Warwick and Salkovskis, 1989, 1990). Such assumptions lead the individual to pay attention to information which confirms the belief and to ignore or discount information that shows the individual is in good health. These assumptions may be activated by factors such as unfamiliar body sensations, hearing about illness in others or information from the media.

The individual's personal and family history of illness and illness behaviours may help to explain such assumptions and beliefs about physical symptoms (e.g. Ehlers, 1993; Mechanic, 1980, 1986; Warwick and Salkovskis, 1989). Various factors include illness as a child, the way significant others responded to their own or children's body sensations or symptoms, and illness or death in the family, as the following example illustrates:

> 'Katherine' was born with a heart condition, which was successfully operated on as a child. Her parents were advised to 'be careful' but allow Katherine to lead a normal life. Whenever Katherine felt even slightly off colour, her parents insisted that she rest and visit the doctor, 'just in case'. She was brought up to refrain from strenuous activities when suffering even mild physical symptoms. As a result Katherine, despite being a healthy child and adult, learned that any bodily sensations and symptoms are dangerous and require special measures to prevent something awful from happening.

Children who are exposed to serious physical illness in their close family, or who are ill themselves as children, are at greater risk of developing somatoform disorders and medically unexplained symptoms as adults (Bass and Murphy, 1995; Craig et al., 1993; Hartvig and Sterner, 1985; Kriechman, 1987; Mechanic, 1980). Themes of danger may underlie the problem of IBS. The client may have a family history of bowel cancer, or have a long history of bowel problems which were repeatedly investigated. Certain types of life events may lead the individual to be vulnerable to worrying about heart disease and to suffer from atypical chest pain, including a personal or family history of heart problems such as mitral valve prolapse or respiratory disease, recollections of prolonged breathlessness in a parent, and witnessing a death.

As well as giving particular meanings to physical symptoms or body sensations, the individual may have a set of beliefs about the self which may predispose him or her to psychosomatic problems. One area may be in viewing the self as bad, and therefore seeing illness as a punishment for being a bad person (Wells and Hackmann, 1993). It is interesting to note the extent of parental illness and disability in the background of people with particularly chronic somatoform problems (Bass and Murphy, 1995), which, as well as specifically influencing the development of health beliefs, may also affect the degree of parental care given to the child. It may be that core beliefs about badness and worthlessness, as are found in people with other psychological problems, develop as a result of emotional or physical deprivation resulting from parental illness; combined with specific messages about the danger of illness, learned from either observing parental illness or childhood illnesses, the individual may then centre the core beliefs around the danger of symptoms (Craig et al., 1993; Murphy, 1993).

A second core belief – seeing the self as vulnerable and the world as a dangerous place – may predispose people to developing psychosomatic disorders and health anxiety. Young and Klosko (1993) describe beliefs of vulnerability, whereby the individual believes that disaster is about to strike at any minute, particularly disease, disability or death. Physical sensations and symptoms are taken as signs of AIDS, cancer, multiple sclerosis or some other dreadful and dreaded disease, and the only way to avert danger is to be alert for signs of illness all the time, worry about any strange symptoms, and seek medical help at the first instance. Young describes how people with beliefs relating to vulnerability to illness are vigilant to anything in the environment relevant to the possibility of illness: the person may either read everything available on the subject of health, or try and avoid the subject altogether because of the anxiety it evokes. Young and Klosko (1993) suggest that the origins of such beliefs lie in five areas:

- The parents felt themselves to be vulnerable, thereby teaching the child the beliefs directly.

- The parents were overprotective, giving the child the message that the world is a dangerous place, and that the individual was too frail or incompetent to deal with these dangers.
- The child either was not, or did not feel, adequately protected; the childhood environment did not seem to be emotionally, physically or financially safe.
- The individual was sick or experienced a serious traumatic event as a child, leading the child to feel vulnerable.
- There was significant illness or death in the family, perhaps the death of one or both parents, leading the child to view the world as dangerous.

Assumptions and beliefs about psychological distress

The notion that somatic symptoms represent a conversion of psychological distress into physical outlets has had a strong influence on the understanding of psychosomatic problems. Some degree of 'conversion' may be common. Many of us, for example, may not realize that some aspect of life, perhaps workload or a relationship, is causing difficulties or stress until we notice recurrent headaches or a build-up of minor symptoms. A more extreme form is known as alexythymia, which hypothesizes that the person is unable to express or verbalize distressing emotions, and so may convert them into somatic symptoms. Alexythymic individuals are said to display a lowered capacity for expressing affect and psychological state. They lack the words for feelings, do not have fantasies expressive of feelings and their thoughts are dominated by details of events in the environment rather than feelings or emotions (Taylor, 1987).

Although it is sometimes the case that people with extreme somatization disorder appear free of emotion, or blame their upset entirely on the physical symptoms and incompetence of the medical profession rather than other difficulties in life, other 'somatizers' have much emotion associated with particular events or memories. Both the lack of emotion, or lack of the individual accepting psychological factors in her or his distress may be more usefully conceptualized and understood as a tendency to pay attention to bodily distress rather than psychological events. This tendency is related to underlying assumptions and beliefs about the relative importance or acceptability of physical symptoms as opposed to emotional ones. This may arise from four assumptions:

1 The individual is unable to find the words to express feelings; therefore, feeling bad will be experienced as physical sensations rather than as an emotional experience.
2 The individual believes that emotions are unacceptable or

dangerous; therefore, the individual will dismiss their feelings and only pay attention to physical sensations of distress.

3   The individual believes themselves to be able to cope with all aspects of life, and to have difficulties is a sign of unacceptable weakness; therefore, the only legitimate way to cope with difficulties is to be ill.

4   The individual believes that the only way to get one's needs met is through illness.

The individual is unable to find the words to express feelings
During our development at different ages we learn through different sensory modalities about our feelings and the relative acceptability of emotions. Distressing and difficult experiences may affect an individual's emotional development in different ways, depending on the age and developmental stage at which difficulties occur (Layden et al., 1993). In older children, information is received verbally and stored in the memory of language. In contrast, very young infants may take in information via bodily sensations such as touch, body position, tone of speech and unformed visual inputs. A number of studies of child development show that infants have difficulty in organizing this stimulation and making sense of it, so it becomes stored as diffuse images or kinaesthetic cues carrying only vague meaning. If these sources of stimulation are difficult and distressing to the child, they can later result in disorganized and only partially formed thoughts, feelings, assumptions and beliefs, which Layden et al. call 'the cloud'. An extreme lack of adequate care giving in the very early stages of life, and emotional or sexual abuse can lead to the development of beliefs about the self, others and the world which are very negative and unhelpful – so-called 'early maladaptive schema'. For example, an individual who has suffered early abuse may believe, absolutely, that she is a bad person. When this belief is activated, for example by the client making a mistake, being rejected in a relationship, and so on, it is difficult for the individual to identify and articulate the distress experienced; instead, the upset may be experienced as physical sensations and symptoms. Feeling bad means experiencing bodily pain, physical symptoms or changes in physical functioning.

This is not to say that all people with psychosomatic problems have experienced extreme abuse during infancy, or that they are unable to articulate any forms of emotional distress except through physical symptoms. Rather, it may provide one means of under-standing research linking early traumatic experience with somatic problems. Women with a history of severe childhood sexual or physical abuse have significantly higher life-time prevalence of both psychological problems and medically unexplained physical symptoms, and greater use of health care resources. People with a history of abuse are 2.5 times more likely than non-abused people to visit a doctor or be hospitalized, and are more likely to have invasive diagnostic tests and operations with normal findings (Drossman et al., 1990). Walker et al. (1993) found a higher rate of severe childhood sexual abuse in women with irritable bowel syndrome compared to patients with inflammatory bowel disease; Barsky et al. (1994) found that adults with hypochondriasis recall more childhood trauma, including sexual abuse, physical violence and major parental upheaval. Chronic pelvic pain has been identified as a consequence of childhood sexual abuse (Drossman et al., 1990; Walker et al., 1988, 1992). For example, Walker et al. (1988) found that 64 per cent of a group of women with chronic pelvic pain had been abused as children, compared to 23 per cent in a control group of women with specific gynaecological conditions. The study suggested that chronic pelvic pain was strongly associated with a lifetime history of depression, and that the location of the pain resulted from the childhood abuse. The authors suggest that chronic pelvic pain may be a metaphorical way of describing chronic psychological pain, and may serve to protect the individual against extremely painful and emotionally charged memories.

Given the high rate of many psychological and personality problems in people who have suffered severe abuse, these studies do not answer the question as to why some individuals go on to develop psychological distress and others develop somatic disorders. It may, however, give clues that if the abuse occurred before the child was able to make sense of his or her experiences through language or images, or the child made sense of the abuse using other sensory modalities, then the individual is perhaps more likely at a later stage to express and experience distress through the body as opposed to the emotions.

The individual believes that emotions are unacceptable or dangerous

'Samia' was sexually abused by her father from the age of eight until she left home at 16. She learned at an early age to 'keep her mouth shut' about the abuse; if she cried, she was told to shut up and not be a cry-baby. When she told her mother and sister about the abuse at the age of 22, she was told again to 'keep her mouth shut' and not tell stories. She became extremely depressed but managed to 'pull herself together' and not think about her past, by deciding to keep things to herself. She was fine for several years. Following a number of difficult life events, she started to experience abdominal pains, with no organic basis. She was told that she had irritable bowel syndrome and that it was stress-related. She was very puzzled by the symptoms, since she was not feeling at all stressed or upset.

Like Samia, a number of clients with psychosomatic symptoms describe their style of dealing with difficulties as 'bottling things up'. This may relate to assumptions such as 'Better in than out', 'If I express how I feel, something bad will happen', and 'If I don't cope at all times, then something awful will happen'. Several studies have suggested links between repression, denial, the inhibition of emotion and lack of confiding in others, and physiological arousal, adrenergic-sympathetic over-activity, somatic symptoms and physical disease (Kellner et al., 1992; Pennbaker and Susman, 1988). Kellner et al. (1992) postulate that the link between repression of emotion and somatic symptoms may not be straightforward, but may operate via depression or other emotional distress: people who inhibit anger are, on average, more depressed and depressed individuals have more somatic symptoms.

As well as individual assumptions and beliefs, there are many cultural factors influencing the expression of emotions. We live in a society where a 'stiff upper lip' is endorsed, and where children, particularly boys, are told to 'be brave' and 'not be a cry-baby' when hurt or upset. Cross-cultural research offers perspectives on how emotional distress is perceived and presented to others, and how the individual, having problems in various areas of life, may convey these in bodily terms. Membership of cultural groups where emotional expression is not encouraged or taboo may also influence the way distress is both experienced and presented (Craig and Boardman, 1990; Escobar et al., 1987; Lloyd, 1989). A research study on general practice consultations showed that people whose preferred language was English were more likely to consult for and acknowledge psychosocial problems and distress than were Gujarati and Urdu speakers, who were more likely to attribute their symptoms to medical causes (Bhatt et al., 1989). In a study of 100 people in Hunan, whom Chinese psychiatrists had diagnosed as suffering from 'neurasthenia', Kleinman and Kleinman (1985) diagnosed major depressive disorder or other depression in 93 per cent; all of the group had presented with physical symptoms including headaches, dizziness and bodily pains, and fewer than 1 in 10 actually complained of feeling depressed. In the local social and cultural context in the mid-1980s, complaining of emotional symptoms came too close to admitting to highly stigmatized mental illness and to dissatisfaction with the State.

The individual believes they are able to cope with all aspects of life, and to have difficulties is a sign of unacceptable weakness; therefore, the only legitimate way to be able to cope with difficulties is to be ill A third theme centres on the importance of psychological strength and coping. Psychological problems such as anxiety or depression are regarded as evidence of weakness, failure or blame worthiness. Therefore, as a response to high levels of stress and life difficulties, such as losing a job, increased workload on individual employees during times of recession, or major bereavement, the individual responds with physical illness, so preventing loss of self-esteem associated with feeling bad (Goldberg and Bridges, 1988).

Studies have indicated that people with chronic fatigue syndrome and irritable bowel syndrome view themselves as strong individuals who are able to cope with all things. The most commonly encountered themes in people with chronic fatigue syndrome (Surawy et al., 1995) concern high standards, and the view that failing to meet these standards would indicate failure as a person or unacceptability to others. Similar themes are found in people with unexplained bowel problems. Toner et al. (1990b) compared the views about the self of depressed psychiatric out-patients with a group of people with IBS referred from the gastroenterology department. Although some of the people with IBS were as depressed as the psychiatric out-patients, they differed significantly in their view of themselves. The depressed out-patients had a negative and depressed view of themselves, whereas the IBS group did not. Other research by Toner et al. (1990a, 1992) indicates that people with IBS have a tendency to hold an ideal and socially desirable self-concept, leading to a need to present oneself in a favourable way. The difficulty in expressing psychological distress may be particularly true for women faced with the conflicts in dealing with career, family and personal wishes, especially when the individual has a tendency to perfectionism in all these areas of life (Toner, 1994). When faced with life difficulties, particularly the challenges of juggling different areas of life and aiming for perhaps unrealistically high goals for themselves, they become depressed; but rather than either feeling depressed or seeking help for their emotional problems, they see the problem as arising from organic, and therefore socially acceptable, factors.

The individual believes that the only way to get one's needs met is through illness The concept of 'secondary gain' is often used perjoratively when describing clients with psychosomatic symptoms. Unfortunately, such views compound the negative reactions of care-givers, and compound the client's feeling of not being understood. Thinking in terms of secondary gain is to misunderstand the client's distress and hints at blaming the client for not 'facing up to' problems. However, understanding what the individual may gain from the physical symptoms can be useful in conceptualizing both underlying assumptions and beliefs and in understanding the maintenance of a problem.

It is possible that certain individuals learn from an early age that one, and sometimes the only way of getting their needs met, or avoiding adverse outcomes, is through illness.

> 'Naomi' remembered her mother beating her and her sister whenever they 'put a foot wrong' and frequently for no apparent reason. Naomi started menstruating at the age of 14, and experienced severe dysmennorhoea. During bouts of pain, her mother would send her to her room for two days and leave her alone. The pain of menstruation was far preferable to the pain from her mother's beatings.

Most children, and adults, will at some time 'somatize' distress, and find that a well-timed headache can lead to a well-earned rest. A child may also learn that complaining of physical symptoms or illness can result in increased attention from parents or being able to avoid unwanted activities or situations (Mechanic, 1980). As well as 'somatizing', many people have a repertoire of other responses to deal with difficulties or meet their needs. It is possible that those who develop psychosomatic problems may not have had alternative avenues of development open to them and may never have had the opportunities to develop a flexible range of coping mechanisms. Assumptions may develop such as: 'In order to get my needs met, I must be ill'; 'When well, I am ignored', or in Naomi's case, 'If I am ill, I won't get beaten'. While at the time, these assumptions are useful, and protect the child from abuse or allow the child a crumb of attention, later on the assumptions are less helpful. Chest pain, for example, may be a way of coping with life's responsibilities: 'Vera', who believed that 'I must not take time for myself: I must work hard all the time' could allow herself to rest when she experienced chest pain; in her case, resting was not a 'safety behaviour' but a means of coping with her difficult job, family and live-in parents-in-law.

Triggers to psychosomatic problems

The third aspect of the cognitive conceptualization of psychosomatic problems is to consider what critical incidents or events triggered the problem. Although these can be as varied as the problems themselves, some general themes may emerge. From the above discussion, it is clear that the triggers to psychosomatic problems may reside in physical problems, psychological problems, or life events or stresses. For example, if the individual has concerns about the meaning of physical illnesses and symptoms, critical incidents may include physical illness, illnesses in friends or family, new information about illnesses from the media or reading medical books (Warwick and Salkovskis, 1990). If, however, the domain of concern is in the meaning of psychological problems, a critical incident may be that the individual starts to feel bad as a result of life events and stresses that make unmanageable demands on the individual. Feeling bad, or emotional problems, trigger an un-manageable threat to the individual's self-concept (Surawy et al., 1995). The triggering events may give useful insights into the client's core beliefs and assumptions and are an important part of an overall understanding of the client's problems.

Are psychological therapies and counselling effective for medically unexplained physical symptoms?

There have been a number of trials of psychological therapies for individuals suffering a range of medically unexplained physical symptoms and somatoform problems (reviewed by Bass, 1990; Creed et al., 1992; Mayou et al., 1995). Psychodynamic therapy, focusing on developing a therapeutic relationship in which the client can explore difficulties, using metaphor to make the link between somatic symptoms and emotions, and helping the client to address current life problems and cope with stress, has been shown to help even those with long-standing irritable bowel symptoms (Guthrie, 1995; Guthrie et al., 1991, 1993; Svedlund et al., 1983). Brief dynamic therapy has also been used to help people with a range of somatic symptoms (Nielsen et al., 1988; Sifneos, 1987). Group psychotherapy has been used to help people with a range of func-tional somatic problems (Melson et al., 1982) and health anxiety (Stern and Fernandez, 1991). Various behavioural and cognitive-behavioural interventions, combining education, stress management techniques, relaxation, cognitive thought challenging, problem-solving and assertiveness training, have also shown varying degrees of effectiveness in IBS (e.g. Blanchard et al., 1992, 1993; Litt and Baker, 1987; Lynch and Zamble, 1989). A further area of therapy is targeted at the fears of losing control and avoidance behaviours, such as using experiments to test out not rushing to the toilet when first noticing the urge to defecate (Salkovskis, 1989) or a paradoxical intervention, such as trying to break wind deliberately in social situations (Malan and Kolko, 1982). Cognitive behavioural therapy has been shown to be effective in helping clients cope with chronic pain (Fernandez and Turk, 1989), atypical chest pain (Klimes et al., 1990) and premenstrual syndrome (Blake et al., 1995). Cognitive therapy is effective in helping individuals with hypochondriasis (Warwick, 1995).

Overall, the research shows that psychological therapies are helpful to people with a range of medically unexplained symptoms. The active ingredients in the various models of therapy lie in helping clients to see alternative, psychological explanations for the maintenance of their symptoms, by making links between emotions and physical symptoms; helping the client see how stress or emotional upset affects physical functioning; offering practical means of dealing with symptoms such as using relaxation; modifying unhelpful thoughts and assumptions; and problem-solving. The importance of engaging the client, and offering a therapeutic relationship in which to re-conceptualize the problem and look for solutions is stressed throughout even the most behavioural of therapies.

3

Key Issues in Working with Clients with Psychosomatic Problems

This chapter focuses on the key issues and challenges to the counselling relationship and the counsellor posed by working with clients with psychosomatic problems. Unlike many people seeking counselling, this group of clients may well not see the relevance of counselling to their particular problems. Many clients will have had perhaps repeated experiences of being misunderstood and contradicted by various doctors they may have consulted and may as a result be angry with or hostile towards the counsellor. Alternatively, the client's agenda may be to get the counsellor on their side in the quest for further medical tests or referrals to specialists. These issues can lead to intractable problems with counselling unless recognized and resolved.

This client group also poses particular difficulties for the counsellor. The client's symptoms may lead the counsellor to doubt whether the diagnosis of 'medically unexplained' or 'functional symptoms' is in fact correct, and whether the client is in need of medical treatment. Clients may bring new and apparently unrelated symptoms to counselling, leading the counsellor to question whether the client needs further investigations. The client may look to the counsellor for a source of reassurance, above and beyond what may be helpful to them. The counsellor may have his or her, perhaps strongly held, views about illness, the effectiveness of the medical system or views that complementary or alternative medicine would be more appropriate for the client. This chapter describes some general principles in working with these key issues. The chapter concludes by discussing when counselling might not be appropriate, and offers suggestions as to others who may more appropriately be involved in helping the client.

Key issues in developing a counselling relationship

Although cognitive therapy is the main therapeutic approach discussed in this book, there is a wide range of models of counselling and therapy from which counsellors come to work with clients with psychosomatic problems. All stress the importance of developing a therapeutic relationship or alliance in which the client comes to understand and deal with her or his individual issues. Issues in developing the therapeutic relationship, such as the basic structures of counselling, issues of transference and countertransference and the key counselling skills for developing the therapeutic relationship have been discussed elsewhere (e.g. Dryden, 1989b; Gilbert, 1992; Rogers, 1957; Safran and Segal, 1990). In this chapter, I focus on the particular challenges to the counselling relationship posed by working with clients with psychosomatic problems. One of the main difficulties is engaging the client in counselling.

Engaging the client in counselling

Clients with psychosomatic problems may be very reluctant to engage in counselling (Manthei and Matthews, 1989). This client group may be very different from those who are actively seeking help for psychological or social problems. The latter type of clients are usually attempting to understand their problems within a psycho-social framework, are usually motivated to consider a psychological approach and, to some degree at least, recognize the importance of emotional issues and are willing to discuss and work with their feelings, social problems or relationship issues. By contrast, people with psychosomatic symptoms may not, at least initially, be motiv-ated to consider psychological factors or recognize the relevance of emotional issues or other problems in their lives. Frequently, the client has not requested psychological help and does not feel it is at all relevant. Some clients may not have been told that they are going to be referred for counselling, and may feel angry and duped when they receive a letter or telephone call offering an appointment with a psychologist, psychotherapist or counsellor. The client's family may have strongly held views about the client's problems. Although some individuals may acknowledge that they are psychologically dis-tressed, they may view this as a result of the physical symptoms and lack of appropriate medical help, and therefore may view counselling as merely secondary to the treatment of their main problems. The client may be very reluctant to let go of a purely physical expla-nation for their symptoms and begin to consider a wider framework. It is not uncommon to meet a black and white distinction between psychological and physical factors, with problems being viewed as either physical or psychological, rather than as a combination of both. There is often a tendency to think that if a problem does not have a known organic basis, then it must be psychological. In a sense, the medical system may compound this 'black and white' way of viewing the psychological and the physical: the more the medical system attempts to purely psychologize the individual's distress, the more the individual has to hold on to a 'physical' explanation, in order to ensure they find appropriate treatment.

Sometimes, a question may arise as to who counselling is for. So-called 'heart sink patients' may be inappropriately referred, to help the general practitioner rather than because counselling would be useful to the client. A referral for counselling may be viewed as a 'last resort' by the referrers, rather than because counselling is specifically indicated. Realizing that the individual has psychological difficulties such as anxiety or depression is often a result of a process of elimination. For example, an individual may consult the general practitioner with back pain. The patient is also facing severe life difficulties and is very depressed, which are no doubt exacerbating the back pains: however, this is not discussed during the consultation. In many cases, the patient will be medically investigated and referred for specialist tests. If nothing is found, then the patient may be asked about other problems. Then, the back pain may be labelled as psychological or a product of the depression. As a result of this 'diagnosis by elimination', clients may have been swept along in the medical system for years before seeing a counsellor. Not surprisingly, some will be confused as to why they are being referred for counselling.

Some clients with medically unexplained symptoms may fear giving the counsellor certain information about themselves in case they are labelled as 'mad' (Creed and Guthrie, 1993). For many people, 'psychological' is a term of abuse and a moral category: psychological is taken less seriously than physical. The suggestion of any involvement of psychological factors may lead the client to feel that they are not being taken seriously, or that their symptoms are unreal and 'all in the mind'. Being invited to consider counselling may imply to the patient that they are, somehow, to blame for their symptoms, weak, and psychologically ill (Surawy et al., 1995). This view is hardly unique to people with psychosomatic problems: it is shared by many in the medical profession, who talk about 'real pain' caused by physical disease or damage, in contrast to the pain experienced when no clear organic basis can be found, which somehow implies that the pain does not really exist.

Many clients will feel angry with their medical treatment; they may, on initial contact, be reluctant to talk about anything else. They feel denied the treatment they should have had, mistreated or neglected. The client's anger can be difficult to manage and contain. The counsellor may feel defensive, personally attacked, or inadequate to help the client after all that she or he has been through; the counsellor may share the client's low opinion of the medical profession and the treatment the client has received, and risk 'colluding' with the client's view in an unhelpful, rather than empathic or challenging way (Murphy, 1993).

It is vital, therefore, actively to engage the client in counselling in a way that does not threaten the individual's view of the self, takes account of their misgivings about counselling and offers an alternative understanding of their problems without either colluding with or rejecting the client's beliefs about their problems. It is probably the case that once the client is engaged in counselling, a substantial part of the therapeutic work has been done. Some of the processes involved in engaging clients are discussed below and are illustrated in greater detail in Chapter 4.

The importance of the initial session and counselling setting

The initial counselling session is vital. As will be described in Chapter 4, the key aims of this session include engaging the client, beginning to conceptualize the client's problems in terms of a combination of factors, and beginning the process of developing a contract or plan for counselling. These aims are met within the context of the beginnings of a good therapeutic relationship, in which the client and counsellor are able to work. The client needs to leave the initial session with an understanding of the relevance of counselling to his or her problems and an understanding of how counselling can help. If these aims are not at least to some extent achieved, then the client may feel very negative about counselling, feel that the counsellor is not able to help or on their side, and may not return for further sessions. It can, therefore, be very helpful to offer a longer session than usual in which the client's doubts and misgivings can be discussed as well as beginning to conceptualize the client's problems and developing counselling goals. This can take up to two hours or even longer. The counselling setting is also vital. It can be most helpful if counselling is located, at least initially, in the medical setting, so that it is seen as an integral part of the client's medical treatment rather than as something different. This can also help the process of collaboration between medical professionals and counsellors.

Listening to the symptoms

The counsellor's main aims in helping clients with functional somatic symptoms, somatization or health anxiety, are to offer an alternative and feasible explanation of the client's symptoms, and to demonstrate how their emotional response such as anxiety, despair, anger or helplessness, and behaviour, such as frequently consulting doctors, may maintain the problems. Initially at least, the client's agenda may be very different. Their view of counselling may be dominated by their perception of their physical symptoms, and their journey through the medical system in the quest for diagnosis and treatment. One way to begin to engage the client is to make a very full assessment of their physical symptoms and medical problems and gain an understanding of the client's medical treatment before looking at psychological and social factors. Asking in detail about physical symptoms, how difficult the client finds the symptoms, how much pain the client has had to put up with, and how concerned she or he is helps the client to 'feel understood'. It gives the message that health concerns are being taken seriously and that physical problems are not going to be dismissed as irrelevant (Gask et al., 1989; Goldberg et al., 1989; Murphy, 1993).

Once the client has been given the opportunity to describe and discuss the physical symptoms and medical treatment, it is useful to elicit her or his own explanation of the symptoms, such as abdominal pain caused by a food allergy or virus, or chest pain caused by spasm in the heart (Surawy et al., 1995). Rather than attempting to challenge these assumptions directly, or replace them with another, equally unhelpful explanation such as 'it's depression', it is more helpful to begin to build on the client's view by intro-ducing the idea that factors which caused the symptoms in the first place may differ from those that may maintain the problem. There-fore, an illness or disease may have caused symptoms in the first place, but is no longer responsible for keeping it going. This begins the process of 'broadening the agenda' to a discussion of factors other than the symptoms.

Broadening the agenda
Once the client has described their physical symptoms and medical tests and discussed her or his views on what might be causing them, it is useful to shift the discussion towards psychological or social factors that may cause or maintain the symptoms and so broaden the agenda (Gask et al., 1989; Goldberg et al., 1989). Most of the time clients are willing to acknowledge and discuss their feelings or social problems and can see the links with their physical symptoms, so long as the overriding assumption is not that these factors are the only cause of their problems. Discussing the history of the problems, particularly looking at what triggered them in the first place, can reveal important clues as to the interaction between physical and psychological factors. Open, exploratory questions and reflections are very useful. Summarizing this information and reflecting it back to the client can begin to open up a discussion of other factors, for

example: 'From what you have told me, it seems as if the chest pains started a few months after a very difficult period in your life: could you tell me a bit more about this time and how you were feeling then?' Reflecting back the client's feelings can begin the discussion of emotional issues and how these may be exacerbating the problems, as the following illustrates:

> *Client*: I want something to be done. I can't go on like this. Why don't you do something: talk to my doctor for me and get him to do his job properly. Would you like to have to put up with this pain all day long?
> *Counsellor*: It sounds like things are really difficult for you and you're pretty angry. You're worried about what might be wrong, perhaps thinking that despite all these tests no one can help you?
> *Client*: Yes, I've been feeling really terrible about it all. I'm so worried that they have missed something, and nobody understands how bad it is.

The discussion can then move on to looking at how the client is feeling rather than simply focusing on her pains and the hopelessness of the doctor. It can also be helpful to look for links between how the client is feeling and the symptoms: for example, 'You've told me your guts feel churned up . . . I wonder if you are feeling a bit churned up in other ways?' may help the client discuss feelings as well as talking about symptoms.

Offering alternative hypotheses

For clients who are very firmly convinced that their physical problems are only caused by serious disease, and who are initially reluctant to consider the role of other factors, the risk is that the counsellor and client get into some kind of 'argument' about the cause of the symptoms, with the counsellor strongly feeling the need to convince the client that they do not have a serious disease, and the client attempting to convince the counsellor that they do. Although it is tempting to try to prove to the client that their symptoms are not caused by serious medical disease, it is both impossible to prove this and unhelpful to the client, in that it rejects their beliefs and indicates that the counsellor is not taking their fears seriously.

Approaches from cognitive therapy for panic and hypochondriasis offer elegant solutions to the difficulties of 'arguing the case' with the client (Salkovskis, 1989). Rather than getting into a debate, the counsellor can offer the client a number of hypotheses. One hypothesis is that the client does indeed have a serious physical illness, and that the doctors so far have not been able to diagnose or treat it. An alternative hypothesis is that the individual is concerned and anxious about the possibility of illness, and that their fear, anxiety and preoccupation with the feared disease and its symptoms is the central problem. The evidence for and against and the usefulness of each hypothesis is reviewed with the client before a decision is made whether or not to become involved in counselling. The counsellor then proposes that they work together for a set time, say three or four months, on the new hypothesis; after that time, if they have had a good try at a psychological approach and the problem has not improved, then it would be reasonable to review their original hypothesis. In this way, the counsellor and client avoid 'getting into an argument' about the cause of the symptoms, the client's beliefs are respected, and the counsellor is able to offer a different perspective without asking the client to accept it immediately.

Negotiating realistic goals for counselling

It is vital to negotiate realistic and shared goals for counselling. Counselling does *not* aim to help the client see that the symptoms are entirely psychological rather than physical. Given that nothing is entirely one factor, and that physical factors play a role in psychological problems as well as vice versa, to simply substitute a psychological explanation for a physical one is to replace one distortion of reality with another. The aim should be to encourage the client to see the full range of causative factors, rather than reinforce the belief that they either have 'genuine' physical symptoms with an organic cause, or that the symptoms are 'all in the mind' and psychological. Unfortunately, belief in this dichotomy is wide-spread, and neither helpful nor a true picture of how we function.

Although the counsellor's goals will be to develop a psychological understanding of the client's problems and help the client see their problems in a different light, the client's goals may be very different. The client may want to enlist the counsellor as a potential ally in helping to get appropriate medical treatment such as further tests and investigations. The client may want to prove to the counsellor that their symptoms are not 'all in the mind', or may regard the counsellor as a new source of expert reassurance (Salkovskis, 1989). The client may feel that the only realistic outcome is to be totally free of their symptoms and entirely physically well. Research in the area of psychosomatic problems indicates that, frequently, clients continue to experience symptoms after psychological therapy but the symptoms are no longer a problem because some of the factors maintaining the problems have been resolved and the client has developed more helpful coping strategies. Therefore, rather than aiming at getting rid of pain or other physical symptoms, it is perhaps more realistic to aim to help the client gain control over symptoms, deal with the anxiety about the symptoms, decrease the disability and limitation associated with symptoms, and reduce the level of unhelpful medical consultations (Sharpe et al., 1992). It is particularly vital when working with this client group to elicit and discuss their expectations about counselling and negotiate realistic goals.

Dealing with medical uncertainty

When working with clients with a range of medically unexplained symptoms, it is not unusual for there to be some doubt in the counsellor's, as well as the client's mind as to whether the symptoms are in fact indicating potential or actual physical disease in need of medical treatment. The following illustrates an example of the kind of situation which may arise:

> 'Eric' is a 64-year-old man with a history of heart disease and two triple bypass operations and constant attacks of chest pain. He was referred for counselling because the cardiologist felt that although some of the pain was angina, much was non-cardiac and likely to be due to anxiety. In the past three sessions, Eric has begun to identify the difference between angina and atypical chest pains, and realizes that his usual response when he gets the pain, to think 'Oh no, another heart attack', only causes him more anxiety and more chest pain. As a result his attacks of chest pain are becoming less, and less severe. However, he arrives at the session 10 minutes late having missed the bus. He is clearly in distress, having difficulty in breathing, and reports that he is having severe chest pains.

In Eric's case, the dilemma for the counsellor is whether or not to seek immediate medical help. If he is experiencing severe angina or even a heart attack, then not to summon help is extremely dangerous; however, to summon help for what turns out to be chest pains brought about by Eric's anxiety about being late for the session may feed into his worries about his health and, in the long run, exacerbate his problems.

Although Eric's story is an extreme one, there are many examples when we are unclear about the meaning of a client's symptoms. This is particularly the case when working with clients with coexisting illness or disability, such as a combination of heart disease and atypical chest pain, or pain primarily caused by a disease but exacerbated by the client's worry or depression. It can also be of concern when a client keeps on reporting new symptoms, apparently unrelated to those that brought the client to counselling in the first place, or where, although the client has a long history of hypochondriacal concerns, he or she may also be suffering from disease or illness. This poses a difficult dilemma, given that, for some clients, repeated tests and medical investigations merely serve to maintain their problems, whereas not to seek medical advice may risk not detecting potentially treatable disease.

Although there are no clear-cut answers to these dilemmas, the following guidelines are suggested:

1　It is important to ensure that all necessary tests and investigations have been completed before starting counselling. If a client is waiting for the results of tests, then it is very difficult to begin to offer an understanding of the problems involving psychological factors as in any way causative of the symptoms.

2　When working with clients with coexisting disease or physical problems, it is important for the counsellor to be well informed about the client's problems, through discussions with medical colleagues, reviewing the client's medical notes or information from medical textbooks. If in doubt, discuss the problems with medical colleagues, without unnecessarily raising the client's anxieties.

3　It is helpful for both client and counsellor to be aware of similarities and differences between symptoms of the disease or disorder and symptoms arising from anxiety or depression which may mimic the organic symptoms but may be subtly different. For example, in Eric's case, he could tell the difference between attacks of angina and atypical chest pain, and wrote these differences down on a card which he carried with him.

4　If a client who is anxious about their health brings new symptoms to the counsellor, a useful question to ask is 'What would I advise this client to do if he or she did not also suffer from anxiety?' The decision as to whether the client should seek medical advice should not be influenced by the fact that the client also suffers from anxiety. There may be a tendency for the symptoms to be dismissed as simply anxiety or to be taken more seriously than normal because of the client's anxiety.

5　Where a client is insisting on further tests for the symptoms or problems that have already been extensively investigated, it is useful to review the original contract between client and counsellor to suspend further investigations for a set period while the client is engaged in counselling. This enables the client's concerns to be taken seriously, while not colluding with her or his anxiety to have the tests done immediately.

The role of reassurance

The counsellor may find her or himself being asked to offer the client reassurance, on a frequent basis. While reassurance from others is essential, it may maintain the client's problems as the following illustrates.

> 'Alice' was referred for counselling for extreme anxiety about breast cancer. She had found a small lumpy area in her breast and had been thoroughly investigated, including two mammograms. However, she was convinced that the doctors had missed something, that even though she had no lumps when she was being examined, lumps had appeared overnight, and that the mammogram machine was not working properly or that they had got her results mixed up with someone else's. She constantly asked her doctor, her friends and her partner to reassure her that she did not have breast cancer. During the first counselling session, she quizzed the counsellor on her knowledge of the signs and symptoms of breast cancer, wanting the counsellor, too, to tell her that she did not have cancer but also not believing the counsellor's view.

When faced with the fear and anxiety of clients such as Alice, it is not unusual for us to want to reassure the client. While offering reassurance can in some cases be part of the support offered by the counsellor, it can also serve to maintain the client's problems (Warwick and Salkovskis 1985). We all need reassurance from others at times, particularly about our health. Many medical consultations, such as illustrated above, are made up of medical examinations or tests followed by reassurance that there is nothing seriously wrong. Most of the time we are able to accept this or, if in doubt, seek other opinions to put our mind at rest. However, problems arise if the individual repeatedly is unable to accept the reassurance, or continually looks to others for reassurance when it may be more helpful for the individual to be able to reassure themselves. Reassurance temporarily lowers the client's anxiety but may serve as a means of avoiding anxiety in the short term which becomes unhelpful in the long term. Reassurance from an external agency may reinforce the client's external rather than internal 'locus of control'.

It is important to work out ways of challenging reassurance-seeking without compromising the therapeutic relationship. If the client has a strong need for reassurance, they may have evolved specific, and possibly subtle, ways of getting reassurance. The counsellor may respond by becoming a 'friendly expert' or agreeing with the client how difficult it is to squeeze information out of doctors. It is important to identify when the client is asking for reassurance, and rather than answering the client's spoken or unspoken questions, reflect on the process and the client's underlying feelings. For example, the counsellor may respond to Alice's questions as follows:

> *Counsellor*: I'm feeling as if I ought to be able to tell you that you haven't got breast cancer. I'm wondering what is going on for you when you're asking me these questions?

Developing trust

For many clients with medically unexplained physical symptoms, developing a therapeutic relationship based on trusting the counsellor may be a key difficulty. Many of these people will have been given conflicting information about their health, or have been told that their symptoms do not have any known or measurable organic basis, and therefore that there is nothing wrong with them. This is, in the client's mind, untrue: they are continuing to experience pains or symptoms, and clearly there is something wrong. Therefore, the individual may have very little reason to trust or believe what others have to say to them, particularly those seen as part of a medical system. The individual may be acutely sensitive to any cues that the counsellor is not taking their distress seriously, or viewing their problems as 'all in the mind'. A number of these people will have little interest in the opinions of a counsellor, feeling that their problems are in the physical and medical realm and that, therefore, the only opinion they want is that of a 'real' medical practitioner.

As a result of these factors, the client may feel sceptical about counselling, and the counsellor may feel de-skilled or that she or he has little to offer. These present potential problems to even beginning to develop a therapeutic relationship and, if not resolved early on, may lead to early termination of counselling as the following illustrates:

> 'Peter' was referred for counselling by a gastroenterologist for help with coping with chronic indigestion and irritable bowel syndrome. He arrived for the assessment session, 15 minutes late, with his wife, both exuding an air of suspicion and criticism. I felt if I put one foot wrong, they would be out of the door and my name would be mud. Peter and his wife both believed, first, that his symptoms were caused entirely by organic factors, and second, that doctors were incompetent in finding out the truth:

sending him to see 'the shrink' was just another example of their incompetence. However, having been given an appointment, Peter had to come, believing it was 'rude' not to 'go along with' the medics. Within the first minute of the encounter, many of his assumptions about his problems and about any possibility role of psychological problems became clear: it was also necessary to address these immediately in order even to begin an assessment. I asked how he was feeling about seeing me. Most of the first two sessions were spent discussing how he felt about being referred for counselling and his negative reactions to the medical profession not coming up with an answer to his problems. In my view, discussing his feelings about counselling felt both necessary and productive to starting the counselling relationship. However, at the end of the second session he reported feeling extremely dissatisfied that we had done all this talking and still nothing had been done. Peter did not attend two subsequent appointments.

Understanding our own assumptions and beliefs

Psychosomatic problems are an area where there are many different viewpoints and ways of understanding an individual's problems. It is very useful when working with this client group for counsellors to identify and understand our own assumptions and beliefs about health, physical illness, the medical profession or factors such as the role of complementary or alternative medicine in health care. These beliefs may interfere with the process of counselling or risk collusion with the client's problems in an unhelpful way. For example, we may believe that the medical profession are rarely to be trusted, based perhaps on our own difficult experiences. The counsellor may have strong views about alternative and complementary medicine, and believe that a client's problems could be solved by acupuncture or homeopathy, for example. It is a fine line between offering a client helpful alternative solutions, and colluding with the client's need to find a 'physical' problem or for others to offer solutions to the problems.

Supervision

As for all counselling, supervision is essential when working with clients with psychosomatic problems. The difficulties and challenges posed to us as counsellors by this client group can be both identified and worked through with the help of a supervisor or supervision group. It can at times be difficult to make sense of the client's problems and understand the relative contributions of physical and psychological factors. At these times, a supervisor can be invaluable. Supervision may be particularly helpful in dealing with the roles the counsellor may adopt during counselling. For example, asking about my feelings about myself when working with particular clients has helped me identify specific pitfalls. When working with 'Nadine', a client whom I was visiting at home because she felt unable to travel, I frequently felt pulled into offering her advice about how to help herself. During supervision, I imagined myself as a 'wise owl', flying in to her home for weekly counselling sessions and perching on her sofa to offer my kindly advice. From this, I could understand her desperation about her situation and dislike of putting up with the uncertainty of medically unexplained symptoms and her consequent need for me to be able to come up with the answers. Supervision is essential to discussing and managing other key issues in working with these clients.

When is counselling not likely to be helpful?

It is important to consider when counselling, particularly short-term, may not be helpful. The counsellor needs to be aware that counselling is not always effective and that other forms of therapy, or supportive containment by the general practitioner, may be more helpful. One danger in working with this client group is that the counsellor becomes yet another 'expert' who has not been able to help the client, so compounding the client's distress and dissatisfaction with health professionals or helpers and reinforcing their feelings that no one can help. A question may arise as to who the counselling is for. So-called 'heart sink patients' may be inappropriately referred, to help the general practitioner rather than because counselling would be useful to the client.

Although there is very little research looking at predictors of outcome following psychological therapy, particularly for clients with long-term somatoform problems, there is some evidence that certain sociodemographic and clinical factors are related to response to psychological therapies (Bass and Benjamin, 1993). Some general rules are that therapy is more likely to be helpful if the client accepts that psychosocial factors affect their somatic problems, and if client and counsellor are able to negotiate mutually agreed goals for counselling. Clients who have long-term intractable health problems and frequently consult the general practitioner and also have personality problems, or clients who are unable to see any links with psychological or social issues are unlikely to benefit from counselling, especially short-term counselling. If the symptoms provide considerable psychological protection, protecting the individual from

Table 3.1   *Factors which may predict success in counselling (from Bass and Benjamin, 1993)*

Good response to psychological therapy	Poor response to psychological therapy
• Younger age	• Pain-contingent compensation payments
• Continuing employment	• Constant, unremitting pain
• Work satisfaction	• Pain not aggravated by stress or anxiety
• Pain aggravated by stress or anxiety	• Long history of unsuccessful surgery
• Life event before the onset of symptoms	• More unhelpful illness beliefs and assumptions about causes of problems
• Presence of reported psychological distress	• Absence of reported psychological distress

more painful, uncontainable or unacceptable feelings, or where there are strong financial and practical advantages to having the symptoms, counselling is less likely to be effective, particularly if short-term. People whose main or only problem is severe chronic pain can be difficult to help. Other factors are summarized in Table 3.1.

When assessing these clients, it is particularly important for the counsellor to recognize and work within their limitations. Some individuals, such as those with long-term hypochondriacal preoccupation with their health or those with somatization disorder, may be referred as a 'last resort' following various other forms of therapy. This does not mean that the counsellor is unable to help, but it may indicate that realistic, and perhaps only small, goals should be negotiated, as discussed above. Referral to other agencies may be more appropriate: for example, clinical psychologists with expertise in treatment of hypochondriasis. Some clients may need psychiatric help: if the client's symptoms have a delusional aspect, perhaps indicative of psychoses, a psychiatric assessment is called for. Family therapy may be relevant when the client's problems are influenced by the culture within the family. It may also be more helpful for the counsellor to help the client's general practitioner manage and contain the client. The general practitioner may be in the best position to offer the client ongoing and regular support, for example by offering to see the individual on a regular basis rather than as a crisis consultation for physical problems. Regular consultations can aim, not to 'cure' the client, but to support the client, manage her or his anxieties and fears about the symptoms and offer support in dealing with other problems. The counsellor, particularly if based in primary care, can work with general practitioners to help them deal with negative reactions to the client, or to negotiate realistic goals with the client.

In conclusion

When working with clients who present with medically unexplained or functional somatic symptoms, the counsellor, from whatever psychotherapeutic discipline, often needs to make modifications to her or his usual practice. Some of the key factors include being able, where possible, to see the client in the medical setting and being involved with the general practice or clinical medical team. This can help the client to express and deal with concerns or fears about counselling in a safer, non-psychological setting. The client's ambivalent feelings must be dealt with at an early stage, and engaging the client in counselling before starting the process of counselling is particularly important. A longer assessment session can help achieve these aims. The counsellor needs to be prepared to 'back off' from some of his or her usual counselling approaches, such as allowing silences or showing too much empathy, as these can be extremely difficult or threatening to the client. The counsellor needs to be flexible, being able to move from a more practical, 'medical' and structured approach to a more exploratory, listening style as counselling proceeds.

PART II: APPLYING THE COGNITIVE MODEL TO COUNSELLING FOR PSYCHOSOMATIC PROBLEMS

4

Beginning Counselling: Issues of Assessment and Developing a Case Conceptualization

> *Patient*: Then what is your secret in the cure of this difficult distemper?
> *Doctor*: I have several: I allow myself time to hear and weigh the Complaints of my patients . . . I take pains to be well acquainted with the manner of living of my patients, and am more curious in examining them than there is occasion for a man to be in any other distemper; not only to penetrate into the Protatartick causes, but likewise the better to consult the circumstances as well as Idiosincrasy of every particular person. . . .
> *Patient*: But you think, perhaps, I am a Mad-Man, to send for a Physician, when I know beforehand that he can do me no good; Truely doctor, I am not far from it: but first of all, are you in haste, pray?
> *Doctor*: Not in great haste, Sir.
> *A Treatise of the Hypochondriack and Hysterick Passions*,
> Mandeville (1711) (cited in Goldberg et al., 1989)

This chapter looks at the key issues in beginning counselling. Every counsellor, from different models and approaches, will have their own approach to assessing new clients. This chapter will point out some of the ways of adapting a counselling assessment to meet the needs of this particular client group and will discuss ways of collecting sufficient information to begin to develop, and share with the client, a conceptualization of the client and his or her problems. The chapter will illustrate the process of assessment and developing a shared formulation, or conceptualization, of the case using two clients, 'David' and 'Evelyn', whose progress is followed throughout the rest of the book.

The referral process and first contact with the client

As stressed throughout the first part of this book, some, but not all, clients who present with somatic problems may be reluctant to accept a psychological or counselling approach and may see the counselling referral as an indication that their problems are not being taken seriously. Being able to prepare both client and the referrer for a referral is a key first step in beginning counselling.

It can be very helpful if the counsellor and referrer are able to discuss the referral process in advance. If the referrer indicates to the client, either explicitly or implicitly, 'I cannot find anything wrong with you, you better see a counsellor/ psychologist/ psychiatrist', then the client is likely to feel dismissed or that the symptoms are imagined, and may be understandably angry or not turn up for the initial counselling appointment. A counsellor working in primary care or in a general medical setting can discuss with medical colleagues the ways they can introduce the idea of counselling to potential counselling clients. It is important that the introduction to counselling avoids giving the message that the client is not genuinely ill, or does not have a legitimate complaint, or is 'mad'. The introduction needs to demonstrate that counselling is an integral aspect of the client's care, with the counsellor and general practitioner or medical specialist working together. One possible introduction may be as follows: Although we have ruled out serious disease, unfortunately we cannot say for definite what might be causing your pain/ other symptoms. I can see how difficult it is for you especially since we cannot help you at the moment (thereby acknowledging the patient's symptoms and feelings, and acknowledging that medicine may not be able to help much further). We have a colleague, a counsellor, who is particularly interested in the kind of problems you're experiencing. Would you be interested in seeing him/her for an appointment where s/he can talk more to you about ways s/he may be able to help? (Bass, 1990)

Being seen to work closely with the medical aspects of the client's care can help the client to feel that they are being treated more as a 'whole person', rather than the psychological being split off from the medical aspects of care. It is also useful for the referrer to offer to see the client again following counselling, so the client does not feel 'dismissed' from medical help.

The first contact the counsellor makes with the client may be via letter, telephone or in person. Whatever the means, it can be useful to indicate to the client that the purpose of counselling is to help the individual deal with the physical problem in question, or to discuss the client's concerns about their health, rather than to 'talk through problems' or to 'help the client feel better'. The changes from the counsellor's usual introduction may be subtle, but can be of enormous importance to the client.

During the assessment and the early stages of counselling, the counsellor has to be particularly alert to cues, spoken or otherwise, of the client's discomfort with or disbelief of the counsellor or process of counselling. The initial contact may be the point at which the client expresses anger or resentment at being offered counselling. The client's feelings must be acknowledged and dealt with when they arise. Questions such as 'How do you feel about coming to see me?', 'You seem to be upset/angry about being here. Can you tell me a bit more about that?' can open a discussion of the client's reaction to the referral. Such questions legitimize the client's anger or resentment, and allow the client to put feelings and emotions 'on the agenda'. They also allow the counsellor to begin to clarify her or his role. The counsellor may like to offer something like the following explanation:

> *Counsellor*: Part of my work involves helping a variety of people with physical problems, like yourself, where there does not seem to be a clear physical cause, and where doctors have not been able to help. It is not unusual for people to find the problems very stressful, which may make the problems worse. And often, people are very worried about the symptoms, which does not help either. Counselling may be able to help with the stress and worry caused by the problems.

Setting an agenda for the assessment

Cognitive therapy stresses the importance of client and therapist setting an agenda at the beginning of each session, in order to structure the therapy and to ensure that key issues are covered (Beck et al., 1979; Day and Sparacio, 1989). As well as these aims, setting an agenda for the assessment session is very important to help the client understand what the initial counselling session may cover and what to expect. Like many others, these clients may not have had previous experience of counselling or psychological therapies, and may have expectations such as 'I'll have to tell you all about my childhood' or 'The counsellor will worm things out of me that I don't want to talk about'. As well as asking how the client feels about seeing the counsellor, it can be useful to ask about and discuss any expectations or fears the client has about the counselling appointment.

The counsellor can then go on gently to offer the client an agenda, for example as follows:

> *Counsellor*: We have about an hour and a half together today. I've had a brief letter from Dr X, and would like to find out more about your problems. I'll be asking you about the history of your problems, and ways you have found of coping with them. I'd also like to know a little

about you, and your background and family. How does that sound? If there are things you don't want to talk about, that's fine too.

The agenda of the first session also acknowledges that the client may not be interested in pursuing counselling following the initial assessment, or that client and counsellor agree that counselling is not appropriate. The counsellor could add:

> *Counsellor*: Part of the session today is for us to discuss whether counselling would be helpful for you. You do not have to decide at this stage, but after we have talked about your present difficulties, I can tell you more about what counselling may have to offer and you may decide that it isn't what you want. If that's the case we can discuss what kind of help may be appropriate: how does that sound to you?

This leaves the decision open as to whether the client wishes to continue with counselling. These initial discussions may take up the first 15 or 20 minutes of the session and are very important in beginning the process of the counsellor and client working in a collaborative way on the problems.

Aims of assessment

Although there are many ways of conducting a counselling assessment, cognitive therapy offers some clearly defined aims, particularly focusing on developing a conceptualization of the client's problems and developing a therapeutic relationship in which to conduct therapy (Kirk, 1989). The specific aims are:

- To begin the process of counselling by beginning to develop a therapeutic relationship, helping the client to feel understood, and offering an environment where the client and counsellor can work in a collaborative way.
- To offer the client a rationale for counselling.
- For the counsellor to gain sufficient information to begin to develop a case conceptualization.
- To offer the client a useful understanding of what may be maintaining as well as causing the symptoms, using the case conceptualization as a model.
- To develop goals for counselling.

Although assessment often takes place during the first session, it can be seen as a stage, during which client and counsellor are working together gathering information about the client and the client's problems, and may therefore take place over two or more sessions. When working with clients who present with somatic problems, it can be very helpful to aim to have at least some shared conceptualization of the client's problems and some idea of the way that counselling might help the client by the end of the first session. If the client goes away puzzled about the possible contribution of a counselling approach, it is more likely that she or he will not want further sessions. Hence, a longer assessment session is very valuable.

Developing a case conceptualization

Although many different forms of counselling and psychotherapy have models of case conceptualization, the case conceptualization or formulation is one of the key principles of cognitive therapy (Beck et al., 1979, 1985). Much of the assessment stage of counselling is concerned with collecting information and developing a conceptualization; however, working with, modifying or refining the conceptualization goes on throughout therapy. A case conceptualization or formulation is a means of understanding the client's problems in terms of both the factors which serve to maintain the individual's problems, and underlying mechanisms which may predispose the client to developing the problems. The conceptualization has two main practical applications:

- It enables the client and counsellor to understand and make sense of the client's problems.
- It is a means of developing an overall plan to guide the counselling.

There are various different models of case conceptualization in the cognitive therapy literature. Most models are variations on a theme, aiming to describe the presenting problem and its maintenance in terms of thoughts, feelings, symptoms and behaviour, and to describe the underlying assumptions and beliefs the client holds about themselves, others and the world. The conceptualization also considers the client's experiences, generally during childhood, which may have led the client to develop such beliefs and assumptions. At all stages, a conceptualization is a working hypothesis; therefore, sharing and discussing the conceptualization with the client and modifying it as appropriate are integral parts of counselling. Useful sources for further information on cognitive conceptualization include Beck et al., 1990; Blackburn and Davidson, 1990; Freeman, 1992; Freeman et al., 1990; Kirk, 1989; and Persons, 1989, 1993.

The general model of case conceptualization is illustrated in Figure 4.1.

Early experience
Information about the client's early and other significant experiences which may
have shaped core beliefs and assumptions.

↓

Development of beliefs about the self, others and the world
Unconditional, core beliefs developing from early experience, such as 'I am bad',
'I am weak and vulnerable', 'Others will always look after me' or 'The world is a
dangerous place'.

↓

Assumptions or rules for living
Conditional statements, often phrased as If . . . Then . . . rules, to enable the
individual to function despite core beliefs: e.g. 'If I am vigilant about my health at
all times, then I'll be safe, despite being vulnerable'; 'If I work hard all the time, I'll
be OK, despite being a bad person'.

↓

Critical incidents which trigger problems
Situations or events in which the rules are broken or assumptions are activated.

↓

Problem and factors maintaining the problem
Physical symptoms, thoughts, emotions, behaviour interacting in a
'vicious circle'.

Figure 4.1 *Cognitive conceptualization*

Assessment skills: curiosity not interrogation

The balance between gaining information and developing the therapeutic relationship can be a sensitive one. One way of gaining
information is to ask questions. However, asking questions does not
mean an interrogation. Cognitive therapy emphasizes asking
questions in the spirit of a collaborative relationship, where client
and counsellor are working together to help the client. One of the
key approaches is *guided discovery*, where the questions aim to help
the client discover new ways of seeing the situation rather than
coming up with right or wrong answers. Therefore, the way questions are framed and spoken is important. It helps to be curious
rather than inquisitive. The counsellor's questions are peppered with
reflections on why the question may be important. 'It can help to

understand anything else going on in your life which may be making your symptoms worse, or may be making you feel upset' can introduce a discussion of social factors or stresses. Throughout the assessment, the counsellor summarizes and reflects back what the client has told them: this helps to show that the counsellor is understanding the client and allows for correction of any mis-interpretations or misunderstandings.

As well as gaining information through questions and discussion, counselling focuses on what may underlie the client's words. There should be a careful balance between questions and reflections. Comments such as 'this is obviously very difficult for you' help to demonstrate understanding. Reflecting spoken or unspoken feelings can replace direct questions: 'You sounded very upset just then: can you tell me a bit more about that.' Reflecting to the client 'the pain sounds awful: it must be very hard for you to have to cope with it all the time' demonstrates empathy and can allow the client to discuss their feelings about the symptoms. However, it may be appropriate for counsellors to hold back on using these key skills at early stages when working with people who present with somatic problems. For some people in this client group, talking about emotional matters or social problems may be particularly difficult. They may feel threatened by the counsellor picking up on and talking about unspoken emotions. Too much focus on emotional issues before the client is engaged in counselling may not be appropriate or helpful. Therefore, offering a structured assessment, with appropriate questions, regular summaries, and avoiding any lengthy silences, can be very helpful in beginning to develop a collaborative therapeutic relationship.

Stages of assessment

The key stages of the assessment are shown in Figure 4.2. This is not a list to be exhaustively worked through, but rather areas that may be relevant to the individual client and which may help to develop a conceptualization of the client. The approach should not be to grill the client for this information, but sensitively to explore with the individual those areas which may be relevant.

Assessing the problems and their maintenance
The initial stages of the assessment focus on the client's somatic problems and factors which may maintain the problems. This stage may take up a large part of the assessment, and is a key stage in helping the client identify what may keep the problems going. The

- Setting an agenda for the assessment
- Identifying and discussing how the client feels about counselling
- The client's main problems and their maintenance:
  - Description of physical problems – detailed description of somatic symptoms, thoughts, emotional response, behaviour
  - Factors making the problem better or worse – situations, behaviours, mood, physiological factors, thoughts, other people, stress, etc.
  - How the client copes with the symptoms, including avoiding activities or situations because of the problems
- History of the problems, including medical investigations
- Information the client has been given about the problems and the client's beliefs about the problems
- Medical and illness history and family history of illnesses
- Mood and general functioning
- Interpersonal and social factors: family, relationships, others' response to client's problems
- Psychosocial situation: employment, accommodation, work and any ongoing difficulties
- Medication
- Conceptualization of the problems
- Developing goals for counselling

Figure 4.2 *Key stages in assessment*

client is then able to distinguish between initial triggers or factors causing the symptoms in the first place, some of which may be unknown, and factors which maintain the problems, which are often the focus for counselling. This stage introduces to the client the idea of vicious circles which may be exacerbating the client's distress or symptoms.

It is useful to start with a detailed discussion about the client's physical problems. As discussed in the previous chapter, this helps the client feel that their problems are being taken seriously, and that their physical problems are not going to be dismissed.

This stage is illustrated by part of a session with our first client, 'Evelyn'. Evelyn is 56, and is on sick-leave from her job as a receptionist. She enjoyed the work, although she found it quite difficult to deal with the pressures of the job. She is married; one of her three daughters is married, but having difficulties in her marriage. Evelyn's mother has been ill for some time; although Evelyn has a sister who lives locally, Evelyn has taken most of the responsibility for looking after her mother. Evelyn was referred for counselling by her general practitioner after she had recurrent chest pains. She had been thoroughly medically investigated, without any evidence of heart disease, as she describes.

Counsellor: Can you tell me about the symptoms you have been getting?

Evelyn: Terrible pains in my chest . . . well, two sorts of pain, actually. One is a tightness across my chest, like I can't breathe properly: I can't get enough air: I've had this one for a while and I get it most days. Then this awful sharp pain, the one that led me to be taken in to hospital: it went right round my chest and down my arm. Then, I really couldn't breathe. I was taken in to hospital then, I was so worried and so was my husband. I had all these tests, an angiogram and I was on a drip for several days. I was in for two weeks altogether – really washed out afterwards. Then, when they told me it wasn't my heart: well, I couldn't believe it, could I? I felt really ill.

Counsellor: Let me check I've got this right. You've had two sorts of pain, one like a tightness in your chest, and the second much more severe and sharp. It sounds like you've had a pretty bad time in hospital as well. Can I ask you a bit more about the pains? How often are you getting them now?

The counsellor goes on to gather detailed general information about the symptoms, including how frequently they occur, how severe they are, what kinds of symptoms accompany the chest pains and other details.

Following a general discussion about the symptoms, it is useful to collect more specific information, focusing particularly on factors which maintain the problems. This can be achieved by asking the client for a detailed description of a recent example of the problem. In particular, a detailed example enables the counsellor and client to begin to identify possible connections between physical symptoms, negative thoughts or interpretations of the symptoms, emotions and behaviours.

The process of working with a recent example is illustrated from counselling with 'David'. David, a 45-year-old marketing director, was referred for counselling from the gastroenterologist, after two years of bowel symptoms. He had been suffering from abdominal pains, attacks of diarrhoea and severe wind for many years, which had become worse in the last year. Despite extensive medical investigations and an exclusion diet to identify possible dietary factors, no medical or dietary factors could be identified. David was very worried about the possibility of bowel cancer, following the death of his mother from bowel cancer. He felt, in view of his family history, that the doctors must have missed something, and that physical factors were the main explanation of his symptoms.

The initial stages of the session with David were spent discussing some of his concerns and scepticism about seeing a counsellor. He agreed to discuss his problems in greater detail.

Counsellor: Can we go over this again in a bit more detail? You've told me you've been getting terrible stomach pains and needing to rush to

the toilet several times a day. Can you think of an example, as recently
as possible, when this happened?

David: Yes, let me think. It was yesterday, I got the pains in the
afternoon and they went on for ages: it only really went away when I
got home that evening.

Counsellor: Can you think back to yesterday afternoon, and imagine that
you are in that situation again. Where were you, what was going on?

David: I was in a meeting to discuss sales figures. It was a fairly informal
meeting, we were sitting around the table, and I had a short
presentation to give to the meeting. Just before we went in to the
meeting room, I was aware of feeling uncomfortable in my stomach.
Then, I was due to speak, I got a terrible stabbing pain in my lower
guts.

Counsellor: [summarizes briefly]. So, the pains were just starting up before
the meeting, but suddenly got much worse. And when you noticed the
pain, what did you say to yourself?

David: I think I just felt: Oh no, not again. There must be something
wrong: this is not normal. Normal people don't get these pains and
don't need to rush out of the room like this: I can't go out during this
meeting.

Here, the client has been able to identify some of the thoughts he
had in response to the symptoms. In his case, the thoughts centred
around two themes: the consequences of needing to leave the room
during a business meeting, and secondly, that the symptoms were
abnormal. The counsellor then explores possible links between these
thoughts, feelings and symptoms.

Counsellor: So, you got a pain, and thought I'll need to rush out of the
room, but that is not possible right now? And how did that make you
feel, when you said that to yourself?

David: I felt awful, sort of stressed. I started to feel sweaty and tense in
my stomach and my head began to hurt.

Counsellor: So, you felt really bad, and stressed. When you felt like that,
what effect did it have on your symptoms?

David: The pains began to get more severe: I knew I had to get to a
toilet, otherwise I don't know what might happen.

Counsellor: [Gently probes to ask more about the consequences of the
symptoms] What did you think might happen?

David: Well, I hate to think: It's not the sort of thing you talk about, is
it?

Counsellor: No, I can see it is difficult for you to even think about what
might happen. Can you tell me what you did next? How did you cope
with the pains and needing to leave the meeting?

David: Well, it was pretty embarrassing. I don't usually have to do
presentations: I've managed to get a colleague to do most of them, but
unfortunately he was away and I couldn't get out of it. It was so bad
that I actually had to leave the room, but said that I had left my papers
in my office and had to get them: I usually make excuses like that. I

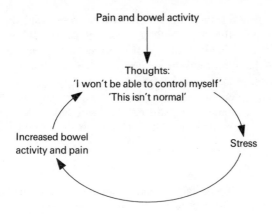

Figure 4.3 *Vicious circle for David*

rushed to the toilet, and came back and managed to do the presentation
. . . not very well, I think. But this can't be right: other people don't
have to rush out of meetings. There's definitely something wrong.

Note that in reflecting back and summarizing the client's experience,
the counsellor uses the client's own terms: stressed as opposed to
anxious, for example.

This example provides a wealth of information about possible
maintaining factors. The counsellor can write down the sequence of
events, so offering a conceptualization of the client's problems. The
sequence is illustrated in Figure 4.3. The vicious circle diagram can
be discussed with the client, and summarized as follows:

> *Counsellor*: I've written down what you have just told me [shows diagram
> to David]. When you start to get the symptoms, and notice them, you
> say various things to yourself, including 'I need to go to the toilet but I
> just can't' and 'this is not normal'. These thoughts make you feel
> stressed, and you described some of the physical symptoms of stress.
> The stress may in turn make the symptoms worse, which makes you
> have more negative thoughts about what might happen and feel more
> stressed.
>
> *David*: Yes, it is a vicious circle, I can see that. But I don't understand
> why I get the pains in the first place.

At this stage, the basic model for factors which may maintain the
symptoms has been identified. The role of stress in exacerbating the
problems is introduced and the way in which a vicious circle
becomes set up can be discussed.

Although identifying thoughts and emotions was comparatively
straightforward in the above example, identifying thoughts and
emotions may be more difficult. The client may be trying not to

think about their fears; asking 'What is the worst thing that might happen?' can help the client to identify specific fears. It can also be useful to identify mental images or pictures the client sees when experiencing the symptoms: for example when Evelyn experienced attacks of chest pain, she had fleeting images of lying in a coronary care unit surrounded by machines, or an image of her own funeral. She found these images very distressing, and would try to avoid thinking about them by telling herself 'just sit down and I'll be all right'.

Triggers and modulating factors

Once a vicious circle of factors maintaining the problem has been identified, factors which may trigger the problem can be discussed, again using a 'here and now' example. David has said that he does not understand what triggers his pains in the first place. The counsellor goes on to explore this.

> *Counsellor*: When you were going in to the meeting, how did you feel about giving the presentation?
> *David*: Well, fine really. I was a bit concerned about it: the presentation itself was fine, but it probably did flash through my mind that I may have the same old problem.
> *Counsellor*: How does the thought of having the same old problem make you feel?
> *David*: Stressed! I'm getting pretty fed up with it.
> *Counsellor*: When you feel stressed and fed up, what kind of effect might that have on your bowel?
> *David*: Well, I guess it does not help.
> *Counsellor*: How do you think the stress might affect you, in your body?
> *David*: I guess it makes my guts more churned up. I know stress can have all sorts of effects, so it is all connected, isn't it.

At this point, the counsellor discussed with David how anxiety might indeed affect his bowel functioning. The conceptualization can then be expanded as shown in Figure 4.4. There may be a whole range of general triggers to particular problems. As well as triggers to specific episodes, David could identify that the symptoms were slightly better when he was on holiday, and worse when there was more pressure from his job. Other triggers and modulators to think about include situations, thoughts, mood and emotional factors, whether the problems are worse at work or at home or at particular times of day.

Coping strategies

It is useful to ask in detail how the client copes with the symptoms, bearing in mind that some strategies may be helpful whereas others

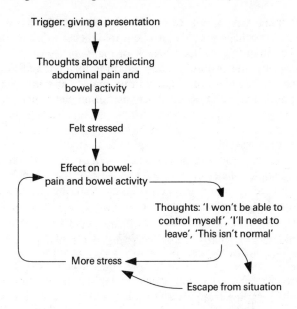

Trigger: giving a presentation

Thoughts about predicting
abdominal pain and
bowel activity

Felt stressed

Effect on bowel:
pain and bowel activity

Thoughts: 'I won't be able to
control myself', 'I'll need to
leave', 'This isn't normal'

More stress

Escape from situation

Figure 4.4   *Expanded vicious circle for David*

may inadvertently make the problem worse. In David's case, he attempted to cope with his symptoms by avoiding certain situations and keeping his problems 'a secret'. Coping strategies such as tensing up his stomach muscles and straining when emptying his bowels in an attempt to control his bowel activity were having a physiological effect on his bowel functions. Evelyn coped with her symptoms of chest pain by sitting down, resting, avoiding carrying heavy weights and not walking 'too far'. This was leading to a gradual loss of fitness and muscle wastage, so that when she did exert herself she noticed more muscular pains, breathlessness and chest pains. Clients who are very tired or suffering from chronic fatigue may rest or sleep excessively, leading to muscle wastage and a number of physical symptoms when they try to be active. Other ways clients find of coping with their symptoms include seeking reassurance, consulting doctors, using medication or discussing the symptoms with friends or family. Alternatively, the client may be overly active, keeping going despite symptoms or leading a very stressful lifestyle, which may exacerbate the symptoms, particularly pain. The significance of the coping strategies must be explored. Clients react to their symptoms in particular ways because of good reasons, and these reasons point to the client's beliefs about the symptoms or their consequences. It can be helpful to ask 'If you hadn't taken that action to cope with your symptoms, what is the worst that might happen?' The client may believe that if they do not rest, they may have a heart attack or incur long-term or permanent damage; or if they do not continually monitor their health, they may miss something of importance. It is vital to explore these beliefs before a client is able to consider modifying the coping strategies.

Avoidance
People with psychosomatic symptoms, particularly those who are anxious about the symptoms, may well avoid certain activities, events, people, places or emotions because of the symptoms. Avoidance can be a powerful factor in maintaining the problems. It prevents the individual from finding out that things that they fear are not likely to happen. For example, avoiding presentations or leaving the room when he noticed bowel sensations may maintain David's anxiety because if he always avoids these situations or escapes, he does not test out his predictions such as 'It's not OK to have to leave to go to the toilet during meetings', or 'I may lose control'. Escaping from the situation is acting as a 'safety behaviour' (Salkovskis, 1991).

General questions to discuss avoidance include 'What have you stopped doing because of the problems?' or 'What would you be doing if the symptoms went away?' Avoidance may be subtle, such as 'breathing deeply', sitting down for a moment to avert a heart attack or avoiding thinking about problems, or it may be more overt, such as not going out. Avoidance often leads the individual to feel less anxious in the short term and can, therefore, be a difficult maintaining factor to change.

Assessing health beliefs and assumptions about health and illness
The assessment stage includes exploration of the individual's beliefs about the cause of their symptoms, particularly any mismatch between medical information they have been given and their own beliefs. For counsellors working in medical settings, it may be that clients will be reluctant or embarrassed to say that they disagree with the medical information they have been given, for fear of offending the counsellor or thinking that it may compromise their medical care. This can be helped by explaining 'I realize that you may well have a different way of seeing things from your doctor . . . how did you feel when you were told there was nothing wrong? What do you think might be causing the problems?' Probability ratings can be used to assess changes in beliefs during counselling: for example, David believed that his problems were caused 90 per

cent by a bowel problem that had not yet been diagnosed, and that stress might play a 10 per cent part in causing the problem. Evelyn was initially 100 per cent convinced that she had heart disease; following her medical tests, this belief reduced to 40 per cent. It is useful to explore the origins of these beliefs: for example, others in the family or friends with similar problems, the experience of being given a medical opinion which later turned out to be incorrect or information from the media.

As well as exploring beliefs about specific symptoms, it is also valuable to gain an idea of the client's assumptions about health, illness and the medical profession. Some of these may be very clear in the way the client describes the problems: for example, repeatedly consulting the doctor with a variety of fairly minor symptoms may reveal assumptions, such as 'The doctors are in control of my health: they should have an answer for everything'; 'I have to always know the cause of every symptom'; or 'Symptoms must mean serious illness'.

The development and history of the problems

As well as assessing the 'here and now' aspects of the client's story, understanding the client's history and experiences and how these may have contributed to the present problems is an important part of the conceptualization. Some symptoms have a very clear onset with clear triggers. For example, symptoms or health anxiety may start during or following a period of stress or difficulties. For other people it can be more difficult to identify clear triggers to the onset of the problems. Some symptoms may arise apparently 'out of the blue' with no clear triggering mechanisms. Asking about life events in the years before the onset of the problems may indicate difficulties that the client has not previously associated with their current problems. It may be useful to go through a list of possible difficulties, such as bereavements, illness in self, friends or family, losing or changing jobs, difficulties in relationships, moving house, and so on. Although there may be a variety of life difficulties that the client has had to face over the past few years, the client may feel that these are not relevant to the current problems because the past difficulties were coped with at the time.

During David's assessment, we discussed possible triggers to the initial problem, and factors which may have exacerbated his problems in the past two years. Initially, David was reluctant to say whether there had been any kind of difficulties in his life. He described himself as a 'pretty normal sort of bloke with the normal sort of problems: nothing I couldn't cope with'. It was clear that some of David's beliefs about himself, such as 'being the same as everyone else' and 'I cope with problems' may have been getting in the way of both David looking at difficulties in his life and his willingness to discuss these during counselling. With gentle probing, and as the assessment progressed, David revealed that he had long-term difficulties with his marriage and with his job, particularly over the past few years of financial recession. He felt that he had taken these problems in his stride and had been the one who coped with the added stress better than most. The situation had now settled down following financial recovery. Therefore, he could not see how stress could really be involved: he had not felt particularly stressed, and now that the stress was over, why was he continuing to get symptoms?

David's history, and how he described it, gives some very important information about possible underlying mechanisms to David's problems. David had to face ongoing difficulties at home and a period of severe stress at work. His style was to see himself as a 'coper', someone who can get on with things despite adversity, hinting at possible underlying beliefs about the importance of control of both his life and his bodily functions. He also had experienced a long time with difficulties at home which neither he nor his wife had attempted to tackle directly, indicating that David's style of coping may be to some extent to avoid trying to sort out problems, and to 'bottle things up' and put up with difficulties.

Medical and illness history and family history of illnesses

Illnesses throughout the client's life particularly during childhood can be very relevant to psychosomatic problems. Illnesses and hospitalizations during childhood may influence the individual in various ways, so it is useful to find out about factors such as the circumstances of childhood hospitalizations, whether they led to separation from parents or prolonged absences from school. A discussion of how illnesses were dealt with in the family may give some clues as to beliefs about vulnerability. What was the child told about illness? Did any illnesses mean instant confinement to bed and time off school? Was the child told to avoid exercise or anything strenuous? It is useful to ask the client about previous somatic problems that may have coincided with life difficulties, such as a tendency to react to life stresses by experiencing nausea or headaches. These patterns of symptoms may begin early on in life, reported as 'I've always had headaches' or 'I was a sickly sort of child'.

The client's family history of illness is very relevant, revealing very real concerns that clients may have about their own health. Many clients with atypical chest pain have a family history of heart disease which understandably exacerbates their concerns for their own health. Similarly, individuals with functional bowel disorders may have close links with bowel cancer or inflammatory bowel disease. Each time a potentially important link is made, the counsellor reflects it back to the client, which helps the client to recognize potential links between somatic symptoms and other factors. A possible summary may be: 'So, you've told me that your father died of heart disease 20 years ago, and last year your brother started to get angina: it sounds like now you're really worried about the same thing happening to you, which makes the chest pains even more frightening for you.'

As well as the 'bare facts' about the individual's history, counselling particularly focuses on the interpretations and feelings surrounding the history. When these interpretations are gleaned, interesting similarities and patterns may emerge, giving vital clues as to the client's underlying beliefs and assumptions. For example, when exploring a client's history of illness during childhood, while the facts are relevant, what the client made of her or his experiences is far more useful information. Repeated illnesses may have led the client to believe 'I am out of control of my body', 'There is nothing I can do to combat illness' or 'I'm a weak and vulnerable sort of person'. However, while the counsellor makes a note, mentally or otherwise, of these kind of assumptions and may reflect them back to the client, it is very important not to try and deal with them too early in counselling, as will be discussed in Chapter 6.

Assessing mood and psychological state
Finding out about how a client is feeling and discussing factors influencing a client's mood is usually the main focus of many counselling assessments. When assessing clients with somatic problems, it is the area which may need to be handled with the most tact and sensitivity. It may be difficult for this client group to identify or discuss feelings. If this is the case, the initial sessions can have a more practical feel, focusing on symptoms and the client's medical history, and how the client copes with the symptoms. A pragmatic approach can be less threatening for the client than discussion of underlying difficulties or emotions. Clients may well acknowledge their feelings of anxiety or depression, but may attribute these feelings to the symptoms rather than being in any way causative factors. This can be a very important key for engaging the client who wants help with the feelings resulting from the symptoms rather than being willing, at least initially, to look at psychological factors which may have played a role in the symptoms' development. Although some clients will have made the link between the physical symptoms and

depression or anxiety, for other clients the link is more complex and not at the top of the client's agenda. It is often best to delay asking directly about psychological factors until client and counsellor have established rapport, until the counsellor has successfully given the message that the questions are not simply to probe for evidence that the client is 'going mad' or that the symptoms are 'all in the mind'. It is useful to ask general questions such as 'We've talked a lot about the problems with your health you've been facing. Can you tell me a bit about how you are generally, and how these problems are making you feel?' This can open the discussion of psychological factors in the context of physical symptoms and can reveal important maintaining factors, such as depression or anxiety about the symptoms exacerbating the client's physical problems. Health anxiety is commonly, but not always, involved in maintaining a range of somatic problems. It is often possible for an initial goal to be to reduce the client's *anxiety* about the somatic problems. This is relatively easy to achieve early on in the process of counselling and, once this goal has been achieved, it is likely that other aspects of counselling may be more effective (Salkovskis, 1989).

Current stresses and difficulties

Ongoing stresses and difficulties can have an enormous effect on the maintenance of somatic problems and the individual's ability to cope with problems. Stress may directly lead to somatic symptoms (Palmer and Dryden, 1995). Stress may make it more difficult for the individual to cope with particular symptoms. In addition, the symptoms may be a cause of stress in themselves. The social environment may be a source of stress or difficulty. Occupational factors may be relevant, in the form of workplace stress or physical symptoms arising from muscular pains caused by a badly designed working environment. The individual may not wish to return to work; the employer may not allow a gradual return to work to help the client to rehabilitate after a period of illness. These factors, and those such as compensation payments and benefits, may play an important role in the individual's recovery or commitment to return to work. Some of these factors can be identified and discussed during the assessment, bearing in mind that some individuals will be very reluctant to talk about these issues until later on in counselling.

Interpersonal factors

It is very useful to ask the client how others are responding to the client's problems and what they think about the problems. Other people can have a significant influence on an individual's beliefs and behaviour, and may satisfy some important needs for the client. We all need help and support from others, but some people may only be able to ask for or receive help when ill. Others may be very worried about what is wrong with the client. For example, Evelyn's husband was extremely concerned about her attacks of chest pain. He would encourage her to lie down or rest when she experienced any symptoms, and insisted on doing all the heavier lifting work, such as shopping, gardening and maintenance work around the house which Evelyn had usually done. She used to walk the dog each day, but he had taken over that role while she was unwell. Evelyn's daughter encouraged her to go back to the doctor repeatedly to insist on another opinion. In her case, the family's response had to be taken into account when considering Evelyn's health beliefs.

It is also useful to consider the role of the individual's symptoms in the relationship, giving clues as to possible factors which may maintain the problems or make it difficult for the individual to change. The individual's background, particularly significant relationships, may influence unexplained physical symptoms in a number of ways. Guthrie (1995) describes a continuum. At one end are people with good enough care during childhood and who are able to form healthy, mutually supportive relationships. These people may develop somatic symptoms at certain times in relation to particular problems, but can recognize the significance of the symptoms and the problems, leading to resolution. At the other end of the continuum are individuals with a history of severe emotional deprivation during childhood, who have great difficulty forming and sustaining mature relationships as adults. The relationships they form may be symbiotic, characterized by a 'carer' and an 'invalid', both having their needs met through the dynamics of the relationship. In psychodynamic terms, the physical symptoms can be seen as an expression of and defence against intolerable emotional feelings. They also help the individual to obtain, from the partner or health professionals, the care the individual needs. These people may strongly resist any changes to the nature of the caring relationships. Some clues about the role the symptoms may play in meeting the client's needs from other people may be gleaned during the assessment phases and may well be a focus for counselling.

Conceptualization of the problems

As described above, conceptualizing or formulating the client's problems is an ongoing process during the assessment as well as throughout counselling. The counsellor draws up and offers the client a preliminary conceptualization at an early stage, as illustrated in Figure 4.4. This helps the client to see what factors may be maintaining the symptoms, and begins the process of linking symptoms with psychological and behavioural factors. The conceptualization also offers an understanding of why the client might be particularly vulnerable to the problems, by formulating underlying beliefs and assumptions arising from the client's early experiences. Although the counsellor may have some idea of these mechanisms early on in counselling, it is often not until later sessions that the client and counsellor are able to put together and begin to work with 'the full story'. The conceptualization for David is illustrated in Figure 4.5

Negotiating goals for counselling

The final stage of the assessment is for the client and counsellor to negotiate goals for counselling. This is extremely important, in that it gives the client a clear idea of what counselling is all about, and a clear structure for the counselling sessions. Clients may be very sensitive to any signs that the counselling 'is not working', and so realistic goals must be negotiated at the beginning of counselling. Goals may be expressed in terms of coping better with the symptoms or feeling better rather than achieving a complete cure. Often, symptoms improve as a result of psychological improvement: the client feels better and therefore the symptoms do not seem like such a problem. The process of recovery may be long term not short term, and counselling may help the client on the road to recovery rather than achieving a 'cure'. Some clients may believe that they should exert 'mind over matter', which is a widely held but unrealistic view: just because a symptom has no clear organic basis does not mean it can be easily controlled by 'forgetting about it', using 'will-power' or 'being strong'. Some clients may be extremely hopeless about the prospects of change, having given up any hope that things might be different. These clients could be encouraged to set small goals for making small changes such as resuming an activity that they previously enjoyed, *despite* the symptoms or pain, or a goal such as 'not to get so low when I notice the pain: try and not let it get me down so much'. One of the goals may be to reduce the client's relentless search for further medical opinions, investigations or reassurance, which may carry significant costs, including the potentially significant health risks and dangers associated with repeated medical investigations.

Possible goals should be clarified early on in counselling with regular reviews to check if the goals are being reached or need to be revised. It can be useful to set a limited time for counselling, during

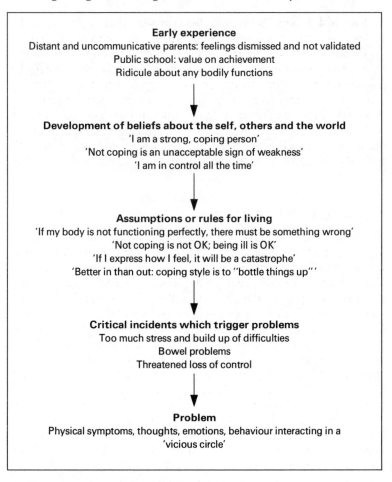

Early experience
Distant and uncommunicative parents: feelings dismissed and not validated
Public school: value on achievement
Ridicule about any bodily functions

Development of beliefs about the self, others and the world
'I am a strong, coping person'
'Not coping is an unacceptable sign of weakness'
'I am in control all the time'

Assumptions or rules for living
'If my body is not functioning perfectly, there must be something wrong'
'Not coping is not OK; being ill is OK'
'If I express how I feel, it will be a catastrophe'
'Better in than out: coping style is to "bottle things up"''

Critical incidents which trigger problems
Too much stress and build up of difficulties
Bowel problems
Threatened loss of control

Problem
Physical symptoms, thoughts, emotions, behaviour interacting in a
'vicious circle'

Figure 4.5 *Conceptualization for David*

which period the client agrees to have a go at counselling and suspend the search for further tests or medical opinions. As discussed in the previous chapter, as part of engaging the client who is extremely sceptical about psychological approaches, it can be useful to ask the client to list the ways of tackling the problems attempted so far, and the relative effectiveness of these ways, such as taking medication, seeing the general practitioner or resting, and compare this to a psychological approach. The client may identify that the present coping methods have not been very effective, and would be willing to try counselling for a set period in order to compare it with other strategies.

Liaison with others involved in the client's care

The initial stages of counselling can involve liaison with others who are involved in the client's care, without compromising the counselling relationship or any agreed confidentiality. Depending on the counsellor's working setting, for example working privately versus as part of a primary health care team or community mental health team, the counsellor may discuss the client with others involved in care, such as the referring general practitioner or hospital doctor. Part of counselling may involve negotiating with medical practitioners not to offer further tests or medical treatment related to the presenting problem while the client is seeing the counsellor. The client may wish to reduce medication, which must be done under medical supervision. The client and counsellor may negotiate that the client will not go back to their general practitioner to ask for further medical opinions about a particular symptom until they have completed the counselling; the general practitioner needs to know how best to deal with the client should they go back on this contract, so as not to undermine the counselling. Other professionals may be extremely over- or under-enthusiastic about counselling, giving the client the message that 'this will help you to sort out everything' or 'don't let anyone tell you it's all in your mind: I'm still sure there's something physical'. It is important to discuss these messages with the client, and if possible with the relevant person. The idea of discussing the client with others can be introduced as: 'before we next meet, I would like to discuss . . . with your doctor: how would you feel about this?'

In conclusion

The initial stages of counselling aim to help the client and counsellor build up a picture of the client, to understand the client's problems in terms of a working model or case conceptualization, and to begin to engage the client in the process of counselling. If the client leaves the assessment puzzled about what counselling may have to offer, puzzled about the model that the counsellor is working with, or angry or upset about any possible implications about psychological factors, it is likely that counsellor and client will not meet again. Therefore, the counsellor can expect the assessment stage to be both busy and demanding. It is strongly recommended that the counsellor allows sufficient time for the assessment, with a long assessment session, and sufficient mental energy to begin to conceptualize the client's problems and negotiate goals. Short assessment sessions late on Friday afternoon are to be avoided!

5

The Middle Stages of Counselling: Techniques and Coping Strategies

The middle stages of counselling build on the conceptualization developed during the first stages, and work towards meeting the client's goals for counselling. This chapter describes some general principles of counselling when working with clients with psycho-somatic problems, and offers the reader some of the 'nuts and bolts' of counselling which are useful when working with this client group. The chapter stresses the importance of only using techniques of relevance to the individual client and carefully integrating them into the therapeutic relationship. The approaches to counselling fall, broadly, into four main areas: ways of helping the client understand and make sense of their symptoms, reducing factors which may maintain the symptoms, strategies to help the client cope better with symptoms, and focusing on other factors contributing to the problems such as ongoing stresses or difficulties.

General principles of counselling for psychosomatic problems

Counselling for somatic problems has a number of general principles, summarized below (Salkovskis, 1989).

The counsellor accepts the client's description of symptoms, pains and suffering as very real, and causing the client distress

Counselling is based on an empathic understanding and validation of the client's physical distress. The counselling fully acknowledges the reality of the client's symptoms, and does not offer a false or simplistic distinction between real physical symptoms and unreal psychological ones. The counsellor in no way implies that the symptoms are 'all in the mind', but looks to help the client understand and cope with the symptoms. Counselling aims to help the client deal with the psychological consequences of symptoms as well as with the symptoms themselves.

*Counselling aims to help clients understand what may be
causing the symptoms, rather than what is not causing them*
Much of medical investigation is a process of elimination: therefore
it is not uncommon for clients to begin counselling saying 'I understand my symptoms are not caused by anything medically serious,
such as cancer or heart disease, but I don't understand what *is*
causing them'. Counselling aims to give alternative, feasible explanations for the symptoms. Any kind of explanation needs to be
relevant to the client's problems, and not simply 'reassurance' that
nothing is seriously wrong.

*Counselling is not an argument, with the counsellor attempting
to persuade the client to adopt a different viewpoint*
Counselling aims to understand and take into account the client's
frame of reference, while encouraging the client to explore
different options. It is often entirely realistic for a client to believe
that their symptoms are caused by medically serious factors, and
to want a definite explanation. Counselling aims to understand the
basis for a client's beliefs, and explores different options, such as
the role of stress or anxiety, or helping the client to accept that
the symptoms are 'medically unexplained' and the implications of
such uncertainty.

*Counselling helps the client identify and test out different
options*
Various approaches can be used to help the client understand factors
which may cause or maintain the symptoms, such as how emotions
influence the perception of symptoms, how 'selective attention' or
paying attention to symptoms makes them worse and how resting
may exacerbate symptoms such as fatigue.

Counselling may focus on coping not cure
Being entirely free of somatic symptoms may be an unrealistic goal.
Counselling aims to help the client to be less distressed and disabled
by the symptoms. Reducing the client's anxiety, depression or
hopelessness about the symptoms is often a useful goal. Helping the
client to develop coping strategies that do not serve to maintain
the symptoms can be valuable. Other goals include helping the
client to lead a fuller life despite the symptoms, making small
changes that add up in the long term, and helping the client not to
get any worse.

- Beginning:
  - Agree agenda
  - Review how the client is
  - Review home tasks
- Middle:
  - Main focus for session: e.g. discussing beliefs about symptoms, experiments within session to test out beliefs, discussing coping strategies, working on other problems
- Endings:
  - Review the session
  - Agree home tasks

Figure 5.1 *Structure of sessions*

Counselling may help clients deal with other problems, such as anxiety, low mood, or social problems, which may be causing or exacerbating the symptoms

Although the initial focus of counselling may be on the somatic symptoms, the focus of counselling broadens to look at other issues of relevance. This is done in the context of a therapeutic relationship in which the client agrees on the significance of other problems, and is ready to look at them in counselling. Although the counsellor may feel that a client's lifestyle or relationships are major stresses exacerbating the symptoms, these should only be addressed and worked on when the client is ready.

Structure of sessions

Although the highly structured approach of cognitive therapy, involving session agendas and home tasks, may be highly alien to many counsellors, as discussed in Chapter 4 it may be particularly helpful for this client group to have a more structured approach to counselling for a number of reasons. A structure helps the sessions to keep focused, so enabling the client to see that counselling is appropriate to their particular concerns. A structure negotiated by client and counsellor helps the client to gain control over the counselling, which is particularly appropriate for those who feel that their health and medical treatment has been out of their control. A structured approach may be less threatening to clients who find it difficult to discuss feelings or problems.

A typical session structure is shown in Figure 5.1. Each session has a beginning, middle and end. At the beginning, client and counsellor agree on an agenda for the session, deciding what they can cover in the time available. An agenda is a way of focusing the

1   Helping the client to reattribute the symptoms by discovering alternative
    explanations.
2   Dealing with factors maintaining the symptoms.
3   Focusing on helpful coping strategies.
4   Dealing with other issues and difficulties.

Figure 5.2   *The middle stages of counselling: key stages*

sessions and helping the client to feel that their needs are being met. The beginning also involves a review of how the client is, and of any tasks or goals the client has been working on between sessions. The middle comprises the work of the session, such as discussing the client's beliefs about the symptoms, coping strategies, working on issues that may be maintaining the problems or other difficulties in the client's life. At the end, the client and counsellor review the session and discuss what tasks it would be useful for the client to work on before the next session, such as keeping a diary of symptoms or thoughts, gradually increasing activities or working on ways of reducing stress. Home tasks enable the client to feel that they are able to help themselves, and not simply at the mercy of their physical symptoms.

Stages of counselling

The middle phase of counselling may move through four key stages, described in Figure 5.2. Although the stages are described separately, in practice the counselling may work simultaneously at a number of levels: for example, helping the client reattribute the symptoms to non-medically serious causes also enables the client to change thoughts or behaviours which may have been maintaining the symptoms, and to begin to tackle the stresses which may have caused the symptoms in the first place.

Stage 1: discovering alternative explanations for the symptoms

Following medical investigations, people are frequently offered reassurance that the symptoms are not indicative of serious disease, but are not offered a feasible explanation of what might be the cause. For example, a common complaint of people with atypical chest pain is to say 'I know my coronary arteries are fine, but I don't understand what is causing the pain'. One of the key aims of counselling people with psychosomatic problems is to help the client to find a plausible explanation of what may be causing the symptoms, rather than what is not causing the symptoms. Part of offering alternative explanations is to demonstrate possible ways that symptoms arise. In some cases, such as irritable bowel syndrome and atypical chest pain, plausible mechanisms for the production of symptoms are available, with reasonable evidence to support the mechanisms. For other problems, the mechanisms are less well understood. Any explanation of causes should start from and build on the client's own theories and information the client has been given. The client may have some incorrect or distorted beliefs: it is a key skill to be able to discuss these and offer more accurate information without the client feeling humiliated or misunderstood. A key skill is not to be tempted to suggest hypothetical or incorrect mechanisms in order to satisfy the client's need for definite explanations: it is more useful to explore the client's need for certainty and how the client feels about medical uncertainty, such as symptoms which have no 'known' cause, rather than offering false explanations.

Making the link between psychological and somatic factors
Several strategies can be used to help the client to make a connection between physical symptoms and psychological or social factors. Sometimes the connections can be very clear, such as somatic symptoms that are clearly worse when the client is under stress. These clients have very often made the connection themselves. A diary, such as shown in Table 5.1, linking symptoms with activities, thoughts or emotions can help the client to connect symptoms with other factors on a day-to-day basis.

The counsellor can help the client to make links by a combination of guided discovery and encouraging the client to test out alternative explanations. A key skill is to help the client to make the link themselves rather than making helpful suggestions. Although it may be tempting for the counsellor to reflect 'I wonder if these symptoms are worse when you are worried/under stress/angry/depressed/', it is more useful to use Socratic questioning and guided discovery to enable the client to identify connections. Making temporal links can be helpful: 'From what you have told me, it seems as if things became much worse for you when you changed your job. Is this possible?'

Discovering and testing alternative hypotheses to explain symptoms
Much of the therapy for people who are anxious about their health involves identifying the client's specific fears and then constructing

Table 5.1 *Diary of symptoms*

Date and time	Situation	Description of symptoms	Rating 1–10 1 = Mild 10 = Worst	What did you do to cope with symptoms?

and testing alternative hypotheses that may account for the symptoms (Warwick and Salkovskis, 1989). For example, a client who consistently interprets her headaches as evidence of a brain tumour can be invited to think about possible alternative causes of headaches, and the evidence for and against her having a brain tumour given such alternative explanations. She can then be invited to test out such alternatives: is her headache worse at certain times of the day or when she tenses up her neck muscles, and better when her mind is occupied with other things, and is this consistent with the brain tumour or another theory?

The process of reviewing alternative explanations is illustrated with Evelyn.

Counsellor: So far you've told me that you are very frightened that you have heart disease, despite the results of the tests and that you believe this 40 per cent. Can we talk about the kinds of things that make you believe that you might have heart disease, then discuss whether other things may be causing your symptoms? First of all, what makes you think you might have heart disease?

Evelyn: Well, I know the doctors think I'm OK, but I'm still getting symptoms, and they seem to be just like those that Jim was getting [her brother who died 15 years ago from a heart attack].

Counsellor: [Writes it down] So, your symptoms are like those Jim was getting: and he died of a heart attack. Anything else?

Evelyn: There's heart disease in the family – it makes me worried for myself, and the fact that I've not been too careful with my diet over the years: that can cause heart disease.

Counsellor: [Writes down] So, there's heart disease in the family and you think that your diet hasn't been too good: can you say a bit more about that?

The counsellor first of all elicits, in as much detail as possible, the evidence Evelyn has for her having heart disease. The next step is to discuss the evidence against the hypothesis that she has heart disease.

Counsellor: You've given me a number of reasons why you think you may have heart disease. Let's look at the other side now, and see if anything else other than heart disease may be causing your symptoms.

Evelyn: The diary did seem to show that I got the pains when I was feeling stressed about things, like listening to my daughter's problems: so it may be stress. Also, the tests did show that my arteries were clear, so I guess that can't be too wrong.

Counsellor: So, the other side is that the pains could be caused by stress and that your arteries are clear. You sound a bit doubtful about this, though: what is the doubt about?

The discussion then goes on to look at Evelyn's doubts about the role of stress and about the medical results, indicating that the 'heart disease' hypothesis has the stronger belief for her.

Asking the client to list the evidence for and against different hypotheses is useful in two ways:

1 It helps the client to consider different explanations for the symptoms.
2 It opens up the discussion of the evidence that the client is using to support the fears. Although, as in Evelyn's case, she may see that believing one hypothesis, such as heart disease, is 'irrational', the evidence against it is not sufficiently strong. Other factors which influence her beliefs, such as how she felt about her brother's death, also need to be discussed.

As well as discussing possible explanations for the symptoms, it is useful to do 'experiments' in or between sessions to test different hypotheses (Warwick and Salkovskis, 1989). Asking the client to hold an arm out and clench the muscles for several minutes produces muscular pain, which illustrates how pain can arise from benign causes such as muscular tension. Tensing up the stomach muscles may lead to changes in bowel function, illustrating how tension can alter bowel activity. Experiments can illustrate how paying attention to symptoms by focusing on them can apparently change the symptoms. Focusing on the heart beat may lead to noticing irregularities or palpitations which the client had previously been unaware of. The client can then be asked to focus attention elsewhere, such as discussing football or describing a picture on the wall in great detail, which may lead to apparent reduction in the severity of symptoms. This can help to provide the client with personal evidence to challenge particular beliefs: for example, if 'funny heart beats' go away when they are not paid attention to, this reduces the likelihood of the symptoms indicating heart disease, and increases the likelihood that focusing on them and worrying about them makes the symptoms worse.

The hyperventilation provocation test is very useful to demonstrate that benign changes in physical state, such as over-breathing, can lead to a range of apparently alarming symptoms (Clark, 1989). Hyperventilating can reproduce chest pain in a proportion of people with atypical chest pain, giving the individual strong evidence that the chest pains are likely to be related to the way the individual is breathing rather than to heart disease or other medically serious causes (Potts and Bass, 1994; Salkovskis, 1992b). The hyperventilation provocation test should *not* be used if the client is pregnant or suffers from epilepsy, asthma or ischaemic heart disease. The client is asked to over-breathe, taking in deep breaths and breathing out as far as possible, at a rate of 30 to 40 breaths per minute for a total of two to three minutes. After that time, the client is asked to describe the symptoms. People notice a range of symptoms and sensations, including chest pains, dizziness, heart racing, numbness in the hands or feet, sweating, nausea or breathlessness. The client and counsellor then discuss the client's experience. The counsellor may ask 'if you had got these sensations out of the blue, what might you have made of them?', leading to a discussion about how the way the client responds to the symptoms is determined by the interpretation that the client gives to the sensations rather than the sensations themselves.

Evelyn, for example, was asked to over-breathe for two minutes in the session. She started to feel very unwell after about 45 seconds. She stopped then and reported her symptoms.

> *Evelyn*: I feel dreadful: dizzy, sweating, my heart is racing . . . and my chest is getting tight. I can hardly breathe [she gasps for breath].
> *Counsellor*: Have a rest for a moment and get your breath back . . . now, just over-breathing like that was very uncomfortable for you. You got dizzy, breathless, noticed your heart racing and started to get a tight chest. What do you make of that?
> *Evelyn*: It's very similar to my usual chest pains only not so bad: they didn't really worry me.

Counsellor: So, the feelings are similar but you didn't worry so much: what do you make of that?

Evelyn: Well, it must be something to do with my breathing?

The test has illustrated a number of things for Evelyn. First, she may be getting chest pain as a result of hyperventilating: she may also be hyperventilating as a response to attacks of chest pain which makes the sensations worse. Second, she has identified that if the pains appear to come 'out of the blue' with no apparent explanation, they are more worrying to her than if the symptoms have some kind of explanation, such as being related to the way she is breathing. This can lead on to a discussion of how over-breathing leads to chest pain and a range of other symptoms. It aims to help Evelyn begin to reattribute her symptoms to causes other than heart disease, and offers her means of controlling her symptoms, by controlling her breathing.

Stage 2: dealing with maintaining factors

Various factors might act to exacerbate or maintain the client's somatic symptoms: the way the individual thinks about and interprets the symptoms; repeatedly checking to see if the symptoms are there; focusing on and worrying about the symptoms; avoiding activities because of the symptoms; excessive resting which leads to loss of fitness; seeking reassurance; or taking medication. Ways of dealing with these are detailed below.

Modifying unhelpful thoughts

Part of cognitive therapy involves helping clients to understand links between thoughts and beliefs and physical symptoms, feelings and behaviours. As illustrated in Chapter 2, the cognitive model of somatic problems hypothesizes that the way a person interprets physical symptoms, or the person's patterns of thoughts that accompany symptoms, influences how the individual feels and what they do in response to the symptoms, which in turn influences the physical symptoms. Therefore, beginning to identify and modify thoughts is a key step in breaking vicious circles which may be maintaining the individual's problem.

The basic principles of the cognitive model and the role of un-helpful thoughts have been described elsewhere (Beck et al., 1979, 1985; Blackburn and Davidson, 1990; Gilbert, 1992; Hawton et al., 1989; Trower et al., 1988). Adaptation of the approach for clients with somatic problems is briefly discussed below.

Part of introducing the model is to do a detailed assessment of a

Table 5.2   *A-B-C triple column technique*

A: event	B: thoughts	C: consequences
Headache	'Oh no, this is terrible, I'll never get my work done'	Anxiety, panic, fear
	'I must have a brain tumour'	Fear, seeking medical opinion, resting
	'Not again, why me, I just can't get rid of these pains'	Low mood, depression, focus on the pain
	'I'll ignore it, try and relax and it will go away'	No significant change in mood; relief at being able to cope with symptoms

typical example of the problem, asking about symptoms, thoughts, feelings and behaviour, as described in Chapter 4. In David's example, he was able to identify some of his thoughts about his symptoms: 'This is not normal'; 'I'll lose control'; and so on. Evelyn could identify that when she experienced an attack of chest pain, she thought 'I'm having a heart attack'; 'I must stop or else something awful might happen'; and 'I can't die here: no one will find me'. Both David and Evelyn could see that when they had these thoughts, they felt anxious. Anxiety, in particular, is characterized by patterns of thinking which overestimate the size and consequences of the danger, and underestimates the individual's ability to cope (Beck et al., 1985). For example, the individual who is anxious about health will overestimate the likelihood that they are or will get ill, will overestimate the severity of danger if it did occur, seeing the consequences of illness as catastrophic, and underestimate their ability to cope, expressed as beliefs such as 'if illness happens, there is nothing I or anyone else can do'. People with pain may have thoughts around 'I can't cope', 'I'll never get better', which lead to feelings of helplessness, hopelessness or depression, and consequent inactivity.

It can be useful to illustrate the link between thoughts and emotions, behaviour and physical symptoms using the A-B-C triple column technique, from Albert Ellis. A is the (activating) event; B is the belief or interpretation of the event; and C is the consequences. For example, a headache may lead the individual to respond in a number of different ways, depending on the intervening interpretation of the headache as shown in Table 5.2.

The context in which the individual interprets these symptoms is very relevant to the way an individual interprets particular symptoms. Factors such as a family history of cancer, long-standing headaches which are difficult to control, information the client has been given, other symptoms which suggest that the client may have a brain tumour, or a brain tumour in a friend or relative will all influence the meaning given to particular symptoms and can make sense of the client's interpretation.

Once the general principles are agreed, the counsellor can ask the client for an example and write down the client's symptoms, thoughts and consequences using the triple column technique illustrated in Table 5.2. It is not always easy to identify thoughts. It is more helpful to ask 'What went through your mind' or 'Did you get an image or picture in your mind when you got the pains?' rather than 'What did you think?' Unless one is a cognitive therapist, people often mix up thoughts and feelings; the question 'how did you feel about that?' may elicit thoughts. David, for example, when asked 'how did you feel when you got the pain?' responded 'I felt like I was going to lose control, like something was wrong', which is, in fact, a description of his thoughts about losing control and something being wrong.

Often the most useful thoughts to identify are those that are connected to emotions: so-called *hot cognitions*. If the client's mood suddenly shifts, or the description of a symptom is accompanied by emotion, then it can be useful to ask 'what went through your mind just then?' These hot cognitions are likely to carry far more meaning to the individual than those which are not connected to emotion, and may in some cases be extreme or unhelpful to the client. It is also important to stress that the client may not want to describe thoughts to the counsellor, and that it is fine for the client to keep them to her or himself if she or he so chooses (Safran and Segal, 1990).

The use of certain types of question can help the client to clarify thoughts. Questions such as what, when, why and how are useful. Sometimes the counsellor can use mental images or pictures to identify thoughts: did you get a picture in your mind of that happening?; what is going on in the picture? It is very helpful to write down the thoughts using a thought record such as that illustrated in Table 5.3.

Once the thoughts are identified, client and counsellor work together to see if there is a more helpful or realistic way that the client could be appraising the problems, one which might help to break vicious circles. Explaining the link between events and our interpretation must be done in a friendly and understanding way, and not give the message that there is a 'right' or 'wrong' way of

Table 5.3   *Diary of symptoms and thoughts*

Date and time	Symptoms: rating of how bad (0–10)	What went through your mind? How much did you believe the thought? (0–10)	Alternative thought. How much did you believe the alternative thought? (0–10)	Action

seeing things, just that there are many alternatives which may influence our reactions to events. Putting the thoughts into context is particularly important: 'Given your experience, it makes sense that you interpret your symptoms this way.' It is vital to be empathic and non-judgemental. Regular summaries can help to check that the client and counsellor are on the same wavelength. At this stage, the key skill is *guided discovery*, with client and counsellor working together in a collaborative way to see if there is a different way of seeing things. It is not a case of the counsellor 'interrogating' or 'firing questions at' the client, or trying to persuade the client to see things from the counsellor's point of view. One common mistake of beginner cognitive therapists is to ask too many leading questions, too soon, without taking time to explore why the client thinks the way he or she does. Questions such as 'Don't you think it would be more helpful if you did x' or 'Do you think this way because of . . . [counsellor guesses]?' are to be avoided. Instead, open questions, posed in a gentle and friendly manner, enable client and counsellor to explore issues collaboratively. A good question to clarify meanings is 'What do you mean when you say x?' This helps to define more clearly the meaning of a thought, which may be very idiosyncratic. Other useful questions are as follows:

- What might be the worst that could happen?
- And if that happened, what then?
- What leads you to think that might happen?
- How does thinking that make you feel?
- How would that work in your body?
- Is there any other way of seeing the situation?
- What might you tell a friend to do in this situation?
- Is there something else you could say to yourself that might be more helpful?
- What do you think you could change to make things better for you?

This is not a list of questions to use to grill the client. Asking questions in a sensitive, exploratory way aims to help the client think about the thoughts and assumptions with a view to being able, if desired, to see things in a more helpful or realistic light. There are no right or wrong answers. The key approach is to use 'Socratic questions', aiming to help the client make discoveries; supplying the answers, making interpretations or giving the client a lecture are to be avoided.

Discussing thoughts aims to help the client come up with benign and more helpful alternatives. For example, the thought 'I'm having a heart attack' when experiencing chest pain can be discussed during counselling, with the evidence for and against the possibility that the pain means a heart attack. A more helpful alternative thought might be 'The pain is caused by tension in my chest muscles: I'll change my breathing to stop over-breathing which will help it to go away.'

Encouraging the client to modify illness behaviour
It is not unusual for clients with medically unexplained symptoms to behave as they would if they were ill. Stopping usual activities is a common consequence of illness. However, this can lead to subsequent problems such as muscular aches and pains, and fatigue. Encouraging the client to increase their level of activity and improve physical fitness can be very helpful, by developing an activity programme. It is important to agree very precise targets, with goals that are definable and achievable. For example, to 'get back to normal' or 'to get fit' may be too vague or too large a target which is therefore not seen as achievable; to 'walk to the end of the road and back on Monday, and one block further each day for the next five days' is a precise target that the client will be able to achieve. A useful goal can be for the client to take up some activity which was enjoyed prior to the illness or problems, and then work towards this goal in a series of small, achievable steps. It is important to

encourage the client to increase activities *very gradually* and in a graded fashion. For example, the goal to take up swimming and be able to swim 20 lengths may start with smaller tasks such as:

1 finding my swimming costume
2 telephoning to find out about times the pool is open
3 telephoning a friend and arranging to go together
4 going once per week, with a friend, and staying in the shallow end doing gentle exercises in the water for 5 minutes building up to 15 minutes.

These goals may seem very small and obvious, but for an individual who has had a very low level of activity for some time, and may have lost a lot of fitness, it is important that the goals are easily achievable and within the individual's limits. Too much exercise for someone who has been resting for a while, for example, can lead to exhaustion and muscle pains. Initially, activity may aggravate symptoms and the client may interpret tiredness or muscle pains after exercise as a sign that the activity is dangerous, rather than a normal symptom of exercise. It is helpful to discuss these attributions with the client.

Any difficulties that the client has in achieving these goals can be discussed during sessions. Often they reveal important fears the client has: for example, 'What if I have a heart attack in the swimming pool?' or 'This is too much for me: I'm damaging myself' reveal continuing fears about the significance of symptoms or the consequences of activity.

For some clients, the problem may lie not in too low levels of activity but in too much activity. The individual may continually lead a busy stressful life, fitting with beliefs about the importance of excessively high standards; the client may engage in high levels of activity when symptom-free which then brings on the symptoms. This can be characteristic of people with pain. For these clients, the reason why the individual is having to keep going at all costs must be explored. It can be helpful to assist the client to work out a more appropriate level of activity, and encourage the client to stick to the agreed level despite the presence or absence of symptoms.

Seeking reassurance
If the client is anxious about the symptoms, she or he is likely to seek reassurance to rule out the possibility of serious illness or to 'put the mind to rest'. Unfortunately, as discussed in Chapters 2 and 4, reassurance may be counterproductive: it may reduce anxiety in the short term but increase the client's preoccupation with the problems in the long term (Salkovskis, 1989; Salkovskis and

Warwick, 1986). The counsellor must be prepared not to respond directly to requests for reassurance, but to try and find out what is behind the client's questions. It can be helpful to ask the client 'What went through your mind?', or 'How were you feeling just now?' Discussing with the client 'What would really convince you that there is nothing wrong?', can help the client recognize that, short of a post-mortem examination, no one can be entirely sure that there is nothing wrong and that most of us live with a degree of uncertainty about our health. It is only possible to demonstrate that an individual does have a medical problem, not that he or she does not.

One way of dealing with the need for reassurance is to negotiate with the client to try an experiment of not asking for reassurance for the symptoms and monitor the level of anxiety (Salkovskis and Warwick, 1986). It may be that, although not being able to gain reassurance is initially anxiety provoking, in the long term the client feels much less anxious.

Medication

A number of clients with unexplained physical problems may take prescribed or over-the-counter medication for the symptoms which may be maintaining the problems. Medical out-patients with atypical chest pain may be on a range of cardiac medication such as nitrates or calcium channel blockers which are not necessary and may have unpleasant side effects. Laxatives can alter bowel functioning and cause abdominal pain; inhalers for breathlessness may cause symptoms of anxiety if over-used. For individuals with pain, there is evidence that the pain may *reduce* when medication is stopped in as many as 40 per cent of individuals. Being prescribed medication 'just in case' may increase the client's conviction that the symptoms are medically serious (Salkovskis, 1989). It is important for any medication to be withdrawn gradually and under medical supervision.

Diet, alcohol, smoking and lifestyle factors

It may be clear from the assessment sessions that a client's symptoms may be related to particular substances or factors in the lifestyle, such as environmental or occupational pollutants, use of alcohol, cigarettes, substance abuse or dietary factors. This is a contentious area and can be difficult to assess with accuracy. Suggesting that external factors may be involved may continue to externalize or medicalize the client's problems when it may be more helpful to look at psychological or social factors. However, there may be links between dietary factors and bowel symptoms, lack of exercise and muscular pains or fatigue, and alcohol over-use and a range of somatic symptoms. It can be useful to encourage a client to examine lifestyle factors. For example, keeping a dietary diary for a few days can reveal links between irritable bowel symptoms and dietary factors.

Stage 3: coping strategies

As stressed throughout this book, one of the aims of counselling clients with somatic problems is to help the client deal better with the symptoms rather than to achieve a complete cure. Dealing with the client's worries about the symptoms, de-catastrophizing the causes, and reducing maintaining factors are all very important in helping the client deal with the symptoms and, for many, may indeed get rid of the symptoms altogether. However, this is not always the case. A number of clients will continue to experience symptoms. For example, a client who has a tendency to experience bowel symptoms when under stress may find it valuable to realize that the symptoms are those of stress rather than anything more sinister, but may nevertheless continue to experience bowel symptoms during times of stress. Although the client may be less worried about the cause of the symptoms, they are nevertheless uncomfortable or inconvenient. Helping the client to be able to manage the symptoms is a valuable goal for counselling.

There are various different ways of helping clients to manage symptoms. Learning slow, controlled breathing techniques can help control attacks of chest pain, particularly when the pain arises from the client's way of breathing putting strain on the chest wall muscles. Relaxation techniques can be useful where symptoms have a muscular basis, and may be helpful for tension headaches, pain control, fibromyalgia-fibromyositis and irritable bowel syndrome. Helping the client to learn to cope with the symptoms by breathing or relaxation techniques can also enable the client to re-evaluate their symptoms: for example, if the chest pains can be reduced by simply changing breathing then the pain cannot be anything serious. Other ways of coping with stress, such as detailed in Palmer and Dryden (1995) can be very helpful in coping with somatic problems.

Whatever the approach the counsellor and client adopt to help the client deal with the symptoms, it must be guided by the individual's conceptualization. For example, learning relaxation can be very helpful in dealing with aches and pains caused by muscular tension. However, if the client believes that the symptoms are caused by medically serious factors, and that one way of averting a possible catastrophe is to relax, then using relaxation techniques only compounds the client's problems. It is more useful for the client to be able to reattribute the symptoms to factors such as muscular tension before learning to cope with the symptoms.

Stage 4: identifying and working with other issues and difficulties

It is often the case that clients who come to counsellors for help want and expect the focus of the counselling to be on issues and difficulties they are having in their lives: issues such as bereavement, relationship problems, poor self-esteem or dealing with stresses in life. It is often the case, too, that these become the focus of concern when working with clients who initially present with somatic problems. Clearly, ongoing life difficulties may pose a stress to the individual, expressed as somatic problems. The somatic problems may be a means for the individual to get his or her needs met in relationships, or perhaps a means of keeping a difficult relationship going. However, the timing and extent to which the client and counsellor focus on these other issues may be very different when working with clients with somatic problems. It is often necessary to work through the above stages of counselling in order to arrive at a point when it is clear that other factors are involved. Some clients may not be willing or ready to look at other issues. For some, the somatic symptoms themselves are the main source of stress or difficulty: once these have been resolved, the client feels the work of counselling is complete. Other clients are ready and willing at an early stage to look at issues other than the symptoms, relieved that their real problems are at last being recognized. Key counselling skills include being able to begin to change the agenda from focusing on the somatic problems to beginning to focus on other issues, in an appropriate and respectful way, without pushing the client into areas he or she does not want to deal with. At times, this is not an easy task.

Some of the ways of beginning to look at other areas of concern to the client are described below.

Metaphors and imagery
In order to begin to change the agenda from looking at somatic symptoms to looking at other issues of relevance for the client, it can be very helpful and illuminating to try and understand the way the client is describing physical symptoms as a metaphorical expression of the emotional world. This is particular useful for clients who have difficulty in putting their feelings into words or difficulty in talking about other aspects of life.

David described his bowel symptoms as 'something inside me I have to keep trapped, as though all hell would let loose if it were to escape: it would be so noisy and messy, everyone would think badly of me'. We explored the possible meaning of his symptoms in terms of other ways in his life he felt trapped. He talked about 'feeling trapped' in his marriage. He described how he could never express any feelings other than pleasant ones; his bad feelings felt trapped inside him. Although he was angry about difficulties in his life, he could not actively deal with them because it involved 'making a noise and a mess'.

Evelyn, during the course of counselling, described her chest pains in terms of 'as though I've got the world on my chest'. This image was extremely useful in helping her to explore the world of pressures in her life, which felt like a great weight. Another client who was frequently being sick, was asked if there are other things in life she is sick of. A client who rushes to the toilet several times every morning can make the connection between the symptoms and rushing around at work in order to try and get everything done on time. A client describing a pain that pulls and twists inside may also feel emotionally torn inside. We have many useful metaphors in common parlance: 'a pain in the neck', 'enough to make you sick', 'feeling churned up', 'feeling like shit', and so on, which may be used to link physical symptoms and emotional state.

Another way of identifying the meaning of symptoms is to see what images the client has about the symptoms. The use of imagery has been developed in traditions such as psychoanalytic approaches and Gestalt therapies. Images can get away from working with conscious, easily accessible thoughts which may have lost some of their more raw meaning (Edwards, 1990). The exercise shown in Figure 5.3 may help the client to make the link between physical symptoms and other factors. The exercise needs time for reflection both during the imagery work and afterwards. It is most useful for clients who readily get in touch with images, can see 'mental pictures', and who are able to get in touch with these and work with them. Other clients find the idea of imagery does not make sense to them, so it needs to be introduced with care.

Methods from other forms of counselling such as Gestalt therapy can be helpful. The 'two chair' technique allows the client to speak to the symptoms and offer the symptoms a voice. The client can be invited to put the symptoms on an empty chair in the room, and listen to what they might be saying. The client can then answer the symptoms, or sit in the symptom's chair to experience what they might be trying to tell the client. This can be a very powerful way of enabling the link to be made between physical pain and other areas of pain in the client's life. The client may bring dreams to the

When the client is sitting quietly ask her to get in touch with the symptoms. Ask how the symptoms feel in the body. Ask the client to allow an image or metaphor for the symptoms to come to mind, which symbolizes or reflects the symptoms. The image may seem strange: this doesn't matter. Ask the client to reflect on different aspects of the image: its size, smell, texture, temperature or sounds. What does it remind them of? How does it make them feel? What is the history of this image, and what made this particular image come to mind? Ask the client to think about the possible meaning of the image in the client's life.

Going back to the original image, ask the client to focus on what would need to be different for things to change. Give this stage plenty of time, encouraging the client to think about what changes there would need to be for a really satisfactory change in the image. Then ask the client to imagine the changes actually taking place in the image. Get them to check on how this feels, and whether this is a good place to leave the image.

Allow time for discussion of what the changes might mean in real-life terms. Ask the client to imagine life having made those changes. What would that feel like?

Figure 5.3 *Exercise to explore the meaning of physical symptoms (Ann Hackmann, personal communication)*

counselling where the physical symptoms may be symbolically expressed.

Working with issues and difficulties

Once the client and counsellor have begun to identify other problems or issues, these can become the focus of counselling. At this stage the counsellor brings into play whatever counselling approaches are appropriate for the client: discussion, reflective listening, allowing the client to express their feelings, helping the client to become more assertive, and so on. The counselling may aim to help the client modify his or her lifestyle to reduce stress. It may be that some of these clients suffer from stress because of having evolved unhelpful ways of dealing with stress, perhaps related to very high standards for themselves and others, lack of assertiveness or needing to avoid conflict at all costs. Various stress or anxiety management approaches may be appropriate (Palmer and Dryden, 1995). A key skill is in being flexible in working with the range of difficulties that the client may bring to counselling.

Problem-solving

Problem-solving is a means of identifying problems and looking for feasible solutions. It has been shown to be helpful for people with psychosomatic problems, enabling them to look for solutions to the issues which may underlie and maintain physical symptoms

- *Identifying and clarifying the problem*   Client and counsellor work together to identify exactly what the problem is, and other questions such as: Who is affected? What are the components of a problem? When do I need to do something about it?
- *Setting clear goals*   The client identifies what, exactly, she or he wants to achieve, and by when.
- *Generating a range of solutions*   Client and counsellor brainstorm what solutions might be possible. The client can also ask others for possible ideas about solutions to the problem.
- *Evaluating the solutions*   The client looks at the list of possible solutions and identifies which ones might be helpful and which can be rejected.
- *Selecting the preferred solutions*   The client ranks the solutions in order of feasibility and selects one or two to try.
- *Trying it out and evaluating progress*   The client tries out the selected solution and then thinks about how successful it was. If the solution was not helpful, the client picks another solution and puts this into practice.

Figure 5.4   *Problem-solving exercise*

(Wilkinson and Mynors-Wallis, 1994). Problem-solving encourages the client to work out practical and psychological ways of dealing with problems, using their own skills and resources as well as help from others. It can be particularly helpful for individuals where life stresses are contributing to the problems, and where the individual is finding difficulty in addressing or solving these problems or is avoiding tackling the problems. The stages of problem-solving are shown in Figure 5.4.

After several sessions of counselling with David, he realized that stress did have quite a lot to do with his bowel symptoms but was very stuck as to what to do with the problems. His general style, he realized, was not to try and tackle the problems but to 'put up with them'. During a session of problem-solving, he began to generate possible solutions to the stress of his job. Once David began to see that there was a range of possible solutions, he began both to feel a bit better in himself and to begin to tackle the problems.

Involving the client's partner, family or significant others
The client's social circle, particularly a partner or family, may have a significant influence on the client's problems. Other people may be a source of stress or difficulty for the client. Many clients have at least one other person who is involved in helping them cope with the symptoms, often a spouse, partner or family member. The other person may hold strong views on, say, the cause of symptoms or how the client should cope, or may be strongly encouraging the client to adopt the sick role (Benjamin et al., 1992). The partner may

actively discourage the client from counselling, being afraid that this implies the client is going mad or that the symptoms are not being taken seriously. The partner may fear that something serious has been missed and that the client should continue to seek medical help. It can be very helpful to arrange a joint session with the client and partner or other significant people, to discuss their fears and concerns, and to describe the counselling approach and goals. Alternatively, the client can be encouraged to discuss the counselling and any agreed goals with the other individual. This can also enlist the other person's help in encouraging the client in between sessions. More formal family therapy may be appropriate where there are clear difficulties in the family exacerbating the client's problems (Griffith et al., 1989).

Specific approaches for specific problems

As well as the general principles of counselling described above, there are various specific approaches which may be helpful for specific problems. For specific approaches to problems such as headaches, sleep disorders, skin problems, fatigue and gynaeco-logical problems, good sources include Bass (1990), Mayou et al., (1995) and Salkovskis (1989). Approaches to problems of pain, common to many somatic problems, are given below.

Pain
Severe chronic pain may have both physical and psychological causes. Cognitive behavioural strategies have been described else-where (e.g. Benjamin, 1989; Phillips, 1988; Skinner et al., 1990). The basic principles are to reduce the amount the client avoids activities because of the pain, to help the client gain a sense of control over the symptoms and to help improve the quality of the individual's life by reducing the degree of handicap caused by the symptoms or by the client's anxieties about the symptoms. De-catastrophizing the pain can help the client to resume activities in spite of pain. Increased pain tolerance may arise from the client increasing the level of exercise.

The influence of psychological factors on pain perception and experience can be explained using the 'gate control' theory of pain. (Melzack and Wall, 1988). The gate control theory proposes that the sensation of pain, regardless of what is causing it, is modulated by certain physiological and psychological processes. Input from receptors in the nervous system is thought to pass through a neural 'gate' in the spinal cord before being passed to the brain. This gate can be open or closed by other activity in different parts of the nervous system. Competing sensations may close the gate, while emotional input may open it, so as to cause the individual to feel less or more pain respectively. This model provides a mechanism by which psychological factors such as our mood, focus of attention, expectations and personality can influence pain perception. It explains extreme phenomena such as an individual being seriously damaged in an accident or during warfare, and having to get others to safety, not noticing the damage until later. The theory also explains why pain sensations are perceived more strongly if the individual is emotionally upset, angry or depressed, and less strongly if the individual is feeling better or is distracted. It can be very useful to explain the gate theory of pain to clients, so as to enable them to begin to exert some control over pain sensations by learning to modulate or close the gate.

There may be a strong association between the development of pain and unresolved difficulties with loss and grieving (Whale, 1992). Sometimes, the pains can be 'heart-felt' as in atypical chest pain, or mimic the site or sensation of the pains experienced by the lost person. When working with these clients, the aim of counselling may not be to 'cure' the individual of the pains, but to help them become aware of the unresolved issues which may have previously been denied. The counselling may act as a catalyst to help the client to see their pain from a different perspective.

Clients with physical illnesses and medically unexplained symptoms

It is not uncommon to work with clients who have a combination of symptoms clearly caused by organic factors and those where the basis is less clear. For example, irritable bowel symptoms may accompany inflammatory bowel disease; people with angina may also experience atypical chest pain. When describing chronic pain, for example, the distinction between 'organic' and 'psychogenic' pain is of little value, since psychological factors play a significant role in all pain, regardless of its ostensible cause. The label 'chronic pain' may describe symptoms caused by organic conditions which remain undetected.

The counselling approaches described in this book can be applied for such people, particularly focusing on helping the client to distinguish between the symptoms exacerbated by psychological or non-serious physical factors and those which are more serious, such as learning to distinguish atypical chest pain brought on by hyperventilation or chest muscle tightness, from attacks of angina, associated with effort or exercise. The client needs to learn to respond appropriately to each symptom. Some further guidelines are given in Chapter 3.

Negotiating for the client to suspend other therapies

It may be necessary for the client to agree to suspend other forms of therapy during at least the early stages of counselling, including the use of complementary practitioners. One reason is that the client may get conflicting messages. Much of complementary medicine involves to some extent a counselling approach, leading to some confusion if different counselling models are being used. Alternatively, the model of complementary medicine may actively conflict with the counselling model, by advocating and reinforcing an illness model. For example, counselling focuses on what the client can do to help themselves and the role of their own assumptions or rules in exacerbating the problems, whereas complementary medicine may 'externalize' the problems by reinforcing the idea that the client is ill and in need of treatment, and so feed into a client's need for a physical-based explanation of the problems. The danger is that the client's beliefs in illness become more entrenched, psychological or psychosocial problems are neglected and the client may be less willing to consider counselling as a valuable form of help. A client with somatic problems who has received little help from conventional medical practitioners may be at risk of spending a great deal of time and money searching for help from a range of complementary therapies, sometimes with little effect. However, other forms of therapy may have a great deal to offer: for example, if symptoms can be seen as related to the client's ways of dealing with stress, then some alternative therapies may help the client to deal with stress. There are some reports, also, of therapies such as homoeopathy, acupuncture and massage helping people with a range of 'medically unexplained' symptoms. It may be more helpful for the client and counsellor to agree on a coordinated approach to other therapies: otherwise the client may simply consult another therapist at the first sign that counselling is not working.

In conclusion

The middle stages of counselling clients with somatic problems can be seen as working through a number of discrete, but often overlapping stages: helping the client to determine what may be causing the symptoms, working with maintaining factors, helping the client to cope with the symptoms, and focusing on other problems. Often, counselling feels like a process of moving from a narrow focus on the client's symptoms, towards a broader focus on external and internal factors which may relate to the symptoms, to a wider stage when the symptoms are left behind while client and counsellor explore other issues of concern. Sometimes, it is clear from the start that the client has very real difficulties which the counsellor feels the client 'should' or 'needs to' work on. A key skill is to pause and not to start opening the Pandora's box of other issues until the client is ready. The pace has always to be set by the client.

6

The Middle Stages of Counselling:
Themes, Beliefs and Assumptions

For many clients who present with somatic problems, a great deal of therapeutic work can be done by the processes of counselling described in the previous chapters. These include helping the client to formulate or conceptualize the problems in psychological terms, make links between somatic symptoms, thoughts, emotions or behaviours and begin to break vicious circles which maintain the problem. Many clients will respond to the theme in counselling of 'changing the agenda', seeing that the somatic symptoms are to some extent a 'screen' for or result of other problems and will readily spend time on these in counselling.

However, this is not always the case, and for some individuals it is clear that their way of seeing the problems, or their habitual worry about health to the exclusion of other issues are key maintaining factors. Although the client may have dealt effectively with one episode of concern about health, or may have reattributed a particular symptom to a particular stress in life, the client may remain vulnerable to future problems. This vulnerability lies in the client's frame of reference or, in cognitive terms, in the client's underlying beliefs or 'schema' and assumptions.

This chapter will build on the cognitive model described in the first section of the book, discussing underlying themes and beliefs which cause or maintain the client's problems. The chapter will describe methods of identifying and clarifying beliefs and assumptions, and ways of gaining an understanding of the origins of these beliefs. It will illustrate methods of revising beliefs, so that they are more helpful to the client. The chapter will also discuss the difficulties of working with schema and the problems that can arise for the client once underlying beliefs are identified.

What are beliefs and assumptions?

We all have beliefs and assumptions about ourselves, others and the world. Such beliefs and assumptions may be thought of as our frame of reference, or set of rules determining how we can be in the world, how we judge situations or others and how we interact with other people (Beck, 1976). Our rules are formed mainly from our early experience, and often become revised as we develop and encounter different experiences. Rules generally operate without us being aware of them. We selectively pay attention to the world around us, screening, sorting and integrating information according to our rules and interpretations. Cognitive therapy makes a distinction between core beliefs or schema, and assumptions. Schema are central, fixed beliefs, often expressed in absolute terms, which develop during early childhood. Core beliefs may be expressed as beliefs about the self such as 'I am a bad person', 'I'm a failure', 'I'm vulnerable' or 'I'm worthless'; beliefs about others, such as 'Other people can never be trusted'; and beliefs about the world such as 'The world is a dangerous place'. Assumptions, in contrast, are often conditional, if . . . then statements, developed to some extent in order to enable the individual to live with particular beliefs. For example, the individual who felt themselves to be a bad person, may develop a rule: 'If I am nice all the time, and put others' needs first, they won't see what a bad person I am', or for an individual who believes they are a failure, an assumption may develop such as 'I must be perfect and in control of everything . . . to make a mistake means I'm a complete failure'. Assumptions and beliefs which may underlie emotional problems have been labelled 'dysfunctional' or 'maladaptive'. In practice, our set of rules may well have been functional and adaptive at some stage in life. For example, it may have been useful for the child to believe 'I am vulnerable' and 'I must always watch out for my health', in order to enable the child to look after him or herself during a period of illness or to enable the child to fit in with the family culture and way of seeing things, and thereby feel secure and accepted by the family. Problems may arise, however, when our rules are not adjusted and revised in the light of later experience and development, or when we take on board rules that are the result of someone else's distorted or unhelpful way of seeing things. Therefore, terms such as 'unhelpful' or 'out-of-date' assumptions or beliefs may be more realistic and less judgemental.

Unhelpful assumptions and beliefs have various characteristics (Fennell, 1989). Assumptions are a set of rules that are learned through experience. They often 'run in families' in one form or another. Many are culturally reinforced, meeting gender or cultural stereotypes which make it difficult for the individual to identify or challenge the beliefs. Assumptions are often unconscious. We are not aware of the rules themselves, only the emotional or physical discomfort that may arise from transgressing them. For example, an individual whose rule says 'I need to be perfect in everything I do in order to be acceptable' will feel excessive anxiety or depression on making a seemingly small mistake. Beliefs are often more rigid and resistant to change than are assumptions and appear from the outside as extreme, irrational and unreasonable. They are relatively impervious to ordinary experience, and are treated as a fact not as a belief. They may be expressed in very clear, simple, black and white language: 'I'm bad', 'I'm weak', 'It's wrong to lose control'. The words may be those of a child, representing primitive and undeveloped meanings which clearly do not reflect the attributes or skills of the individual. They are often unhelpful and not functional, preventing the individual achieving goals in life.

Deeply held beliefs and assumptions exert an ongoing influence on how we perceive and behave in our worlds. An individual who believes, for example, 'I am a failure', may have many examples throughout life to prove that this belief is distorted; however, we have subtle ways of discounting and ignoring information which does not confirm our beliefs while collecting and remembering instances where the belief is confirmed. Young (1990) describes the process of 'schema maintenance', whereby our beliefs become self-fulfilling prophesies, and we pay attention to information or behave in a manner which confirms our beliefs and discount, ignore or alter information which disconfirms the belief. The process has been compared to that of a prejudice (Padesky, 1993). A person who believes 'I am weak and vulnerable' will remember the times of illness or weakness and forget or discount the times when the individual was well or able to cope alone. The belief also means that the individual does not go into situations where the belief may be challenged: for example, always 'taking care', never exerting themself, taking an 'easy job' and never going too far from home. An example of the maintenance of a belief about vulnerability can be seen in the story of Colin in Frances Hodgson Burnett's *The Secret Garden*. Colin's father, having lost his wife, believed that he was vulnerable to losing his son. Colin, in turn, was brought up with the powerful belief that he was weak, vulnerable, ill and about to die. He behaved as an invalid, and many different symptoms were taken as evidence that he was ill. Having spent most of his life in bed, he naturally became weak and unable to do much for himself: therefore, when he attempted to get out of bed, he experienced weakness and muscle pains. These in turn were taken by himself, by his father and by his nurses as confirmation of illness. His belief 'I am weak and vulnerable' was therefore constantly confirmed: until he was rescued from his plight by the young heroine, Mary, who refused to believe or endorse Colin's schema.

Types of unhelpful assumptions underlying psychosomatic problems

Unhelpful assumptions often fit into three areas: achievement, acceptance and control (Beck et al., 1985). Of particular relevance to clients with health issues may be the issue of control: feeling out of control of one's body, expecting or allowing medical practitioners to have control over the individual's health, or excessive concern about being out of control of emotions or bodily states. Two areas of assumptions and beliefs are outlined in Chapter 2: assumptions about the meaning of physical symptoms, and assumptions about the meaning of psychological distress. This is not to say that these are the only kinds of assumptions underlying somatic problems and they should not be used as any kind of horoscope to forecast problems. Individuals have a whole range of idiosyncratic assumptions and beliefs, some of which may operate more than others depending on individual circumstances or situations. However, it is valuable to bear in mind the kinds of area which may be of concern to the individual, in order to be able to identify a possible assumption when it is in action, and to be able to begin to help the client to identify and work with the set of rules.

Key issues and skills in working with assumptions

Identifying and working with clients' assumptions are helpful for a number of reasons. Unhelpful assumptions leave the client vulnerable to the risk of relapse: although counselling may help the client deal with and work through the present episode of the problem, unless the rules underlying the problem are also worked through, the client may experience similar problems in future. Working with assumptions helps the client to develop skills to deal with future problems.

Understanding the client's frame of reference is central to many different schools of counselling. When working with assumptions and core beliefs from the perspective of cognitive therapy, many of the counselling skills used are the same as those employed in many forms of counselling. Cognitive therapy in particular emphasizes working in a way that is explicit and collaborative: the client's rules are openly described, verbalized and examined as though they are hypotheses about the world rather than absolute rules (Beck et al., 1990; Young, 1990; Young and Klosko, 1993). Work with assumptions and beliefs requires a number of key skills and approaches. Despite all the drawbacks and difficulties our set of rules may pose, our assumptions and beliefs are very central to our frame of reference, fitting like a comfortable old pair of slippers. They feel right, and to act or think against them may seem dangerous and anxiety-provoking. It can, therefore, be very threatening to have these beliefs exposed or challenged, and can imply to the client that they have 'got it wrong', sometimes over many years. Therefore, the counsellor needs to proceed with empathy and sensitivity, and work with, not against, the client. There should be no sense that some beliefs are 'right' and others are 'wrong', or a sense of the client and counsellor getting into an argument: the counsellor's task is to understand the client's viewpoint however much the counsellor may disagree with it or see it as irrational. Should there be a sense of counsellor and client arguing against each other, the focus should become the counselling process not the relative merits of each view. The counsellor must work at the client's own pace and be sensitive to cues, spoken or unspoken, that the client is uncomfortable with the process of counselling.

Identifying assumptions and beliefs

The information for identifying a client's beliefs and assumptions comes from many sources (Fennell, 1989):

- *Themes which emerge during counselling*, for example, David had a strong theme of needing to be in control expressed as a fear of losing control of his bowels, of his life and of his feelings.
- *Patterns in the clients way of thinking*, for example, the thought 'This is serious: I might die' in response to relatively minor physical symptoms may indicate an assumption such as 'All physical symptoms may indicate serious disease' or 'I'm vulnerable where others are strong'.
- *Global evaluations of the self or others*, for example, labelling the self as 'Always in control', 'A weakling', or labelling others such as 'All doctors are completely wrong'.
- *Memories or family sayings*, such as 'My sister was the strong one: I was the sickly one', or 'We're a family of achievers'. Specific memories may point to assumptions, such as memories of illness or parental separations.
- *Highs or lows of mood* may indicate that a rule has been met or violated. For example, if the client becomes extremely anxious about not being able to get an urgent appointment with the doctor for seemingly minor symptoms, this may point to an assumption such as 'If anything is wrong, I must always seek medical advice as soon as possible'.
- *The client's response to counselling* or to the counsellor also points strongly to the client's rules.

The downward arrow technique (Burns, 1980) can be used to identify a client's underlying assumptions or rules. This involves a series of questions to find out the meaning behind the client's words. Questions may include:

- What might happen if . . . ?
- Suppose what you say is true: what would that mean to you?
- What would be so bad, for you, if that did happen?
- What is the worst that could happen?
- And if that happened, what would that say about you, others or the world?

An example of the downward arrow technique as used with David is given below.

> *Counsellor*: You said that it would be terrible if you were to have to leave a meeting in order to rush to the toilet. What would be so bad, for you, about having to do that?
>
> *David*: Everyone would notice. It's just not the done thing, is it?
>
> *Counsellor*: Suppose that was true: what would that mean to you, everyone noticing and you not doing the done thing?
>
> *David*: They'd think badly of me: they'd think I wasn't in control of myself.
>
> *Counsellor*: And if that was the case, other people thinking that you're not in control of yourself: what would that mean?
>
> *David*: It would mean that I'm not in control.
>
> *Counsellor*: What's the worst that might happen, if you're not in control?
>
> *David*: I'd probably lose everything: I'd lose their respect, I'd be a bit of a failure.
>
> *Counsellor*: Is there a rule here?
>
> *David*: I guess I have to be in control: I'll lose others' respect and be a failure if I'm not in control. That's what my rule is telling me.

The downward arrow approach involves peeling away the layers of meaning to identify what is beneath the client's specific fears or symptoms. The questions can be repeated several times until a 'bottom line' is reached. In David's case, being a 'failure' was the bottom line: he had to protect himself from feeling a failure by maintaining strict control of himself.

Using imagery to identify assumptions

Verbal discussion cannot always reach assumptions or rules, particularly when the assumptions are charged with emotion, or if the individual has an intellectualizing style or avoids emotion by excessive talking. Working with the client's images can be a powerful way of identifying meanings to the individual (Edwards, 1990; Wells and Hackmann, 1993). Images are often far more charged

- What is so bad about the events in the image?
- What does that mean to you?
- What is the worst that can happen?
- How do you feel right now, emotionally and in terms of body sensations in the image?
- How did you get into this situation?
- What is going through your mind in the image right now?
- Does the image remind you of anything? What are your earliest memories of the feelings/thoughts/sensations/experiences in the image? Where were you? How old were you? What was happening in your life at the time? How did you feel about yourself at that time? What does that mean?

Figure 6.1 *Questions to explore imagery (from Wells and Hackmann, 1993)*

with meaning than are words and, therefore, give more clues as to underlying assumptions.

Ways of getting in touch with images include asking 'Did you have a picture in your mind just then?' Once the individual has come up with an image, the client can be asked to describe it in greater detail. Questions such as 'What is happening? Who else is in the image? What are they doing or saying?' can help the client to be more specific about the image. Once the image is identified, the types of questions shown in Figure 6.1 can be used to help the client to unpack the image and explore its personal meaning, implications and origins.

The images can give vital clues as to the individual's underlying rules and beliefs and also about the origins of the beliefs. For example, for David, his fear of losing control meant that he found it very difficult to express his feelings. We used imagery to try and uncover the meaning behind expressing himself.

Counsellor: What would it mean to you to say how you were feeling? Can you form an image of what would happen if you were to let your emotions out?

David: I can see myself completely losing control. The words just coming blurting out of me; all over the place, people freezing as they stare at me in shock and disbelief: I'm running out of the room screaming. I'd lose my job. I'll lose everything, and I'd be a long way down the ladder.

Counsellor: And then what might happen? Do you get a picture of that?

David: I see myself being extremely isolated and lonely, sitting in an empty room, all alone . . . a real failure.

Counsellor: So, what you're saying is to express things has disastrous consequences . . . a complete loss of everything, making you a complete failure.

Using metaphor to explore assumptions

Assumptions may also be explored by using metaphor. The aim is for the counsellor and client to identify a symbol or metaphor representing the symptoms, and then explore the meaning of the symbol. Evelyn described her symptoms as a 'heaviness on her chest' or a 'weight'. Her metaphor for the symptoms was 'I've got the world on my chest'. She could then go on to describe what the world was made up of: she could see 'continents' of problems – her mother, her daughter, her job, her neighbour who deluged her with her problems, and so on. By supporting the world on her chest she saw herself as the strong person who could take on board all these problems; however, she could also see that 'being ill' with chest pains was a way of letting go of the world for a while. The metaphor enabled Evelyn to describe some of her beliefs and assumptions: 'I must cope with the world'; 'I'm responsible'; 'If others have problems it's my job to hold them up'; and 'It's only OK to say no to others when I'm ill'.

Modifying and revising assumptions

For some clients, simply identifying the rules enables the client to begin to change. Once articulated, the client may well be able to see that it is not realistic or helpful to hold such extreme black and white views. The counsellor can encourage the client to look at the grey area between the black and white extremes posed by the assumption. The assumption may be seen to be an ideal, or a preference, rather than an absolute necessity. For example, although it may be preferable to be well all the time, or always free of symptoms, perfect at everything and always in control, it is also unrealistic and impossible to achieve. To be imperfect, symptom-laden, suffering the aches and pains of life and age, and making a mess of things sometimes is to be human rather than a disaster. Evelyn, for example, was not fully aware of how much she subordinated herself to others: once she was able to articulate her assumptions, she began to see how unfair and unhelpful they were to her.

Working with assumptions is similar to the approaches described in the previous chapter to challenge thoughts. Some key questions that the counsellor and client may discuss in order to challenge assumptions are shown in Figure 6.2. David, for example, could see that his need to be in control and not cause an explosion had served him well in several ways. It had enabled him to stay with his wife, despite their difficulties, and so give their children a secure base, which he felt was important. He had also done well in his career, and still had a steady job at a time when many of his colleagues

- What is the assumption? What are my exact words to describe the rule.
- In what way has this rule affected me? What areas of life has it affected, e.g. school, work, relationships, leisure, domestic life?
- Where did the rule come from? What experiences contributed to its development? Rules make a lot of sense when first developed, but may need revision in the light of subsequent, or adult, experience.
- What are its pros and cons? What would I risk if I gave it up?
- In what ways is the rule unreasonable? In what ways is it a distortion of reality? What are the ways it is helping or hindering me?
- What would be a more helpful and realistic alternative, one that would give me the pay-offs and avoid the disadvantages? Is there another way of seeing things, which is more flexible, more realistic and more helpful, giving me the advantages of the assumption without the costs?
- What do I need to do to change the rule?

Figure 6.2 *Questions to help the client discover alternative assumptions (from Beck et al., 1979, 1985; Burns, 1980)*

were facing difficulties at work. However, he could see the disadvantages of his rules. He felt that he had not tackled problems that needed to be tackled, so leaving things longer and therefore potentially making them more difficult to solve. He felt that being in control and not showing his feelings made him a rather boring person and left him socially isolated. He also could see that he was suffering from physical symptoms as a result.

Using images to modify assumptions
Clients who are able to 'think in pictures' and identify clear images, and who are able to work with such images, may find it helpful to use imagery to modify assumptions. Although several texts on visualization suggest that substituting a positive ending is a means of changing images, in cognitive terms this may be counterproductive since merely looking at a 'happy ending' enables the client to avoid looking at the feared catastrophes or consequences of the image, and may actually prevent the client from re-evaluating the image and coming up with a more appropriate alternative. Very often people freeze the image in time and do not look beyond. Being able to examine the image may help the client to modify it, by projecting the image in time, or by re-evaluating the reality of the image. Ways of working with images are described by Edwards (1990). David, for example, could only see complete catastrophe arising from him expressing his feelings or needing to leave a room rapidly in order to use the toilet. Once he could project his image forward in time, he could see that not many people would in fact notice his behaviour,

and even if they did, they would forget it in a few minutes. He was able to begin to change his assumption from 'It is terrible to lose control' to 'Even if I did lose control, nothing serious would or could happen'.

Images also enable the client to identify and get in touch with relevant childhood experiences which may have influence on the assumptions. David moved from his image of rushing out of his workplace and an earlier childhood memory of having a bad stomach upset as a child and having to rush out of his class. He felt very embarrassed and was subsequently teased by his peers for weeks afterwards, leaving him humiliated and upset. When a client identifies a relevant childhood memory, it is helpful to ask the client what beliefs he or she would have been operating at that time. David could identify his belief as 'I must be in control: otherwise I'll be rejected and humiliated'. The conceptualization of the belief may take time to be put together in a meaningful way. The client may regress in the session and become the age she or he was during the memory, and therefore find it difficult to articulate the meaning of the memory. The client can be invited to re-evaluate the image or memory from an adult perspective.

Challenging assumptions: taking risks
One powerful way of testing out rules is to devise experiments in which the individual does not act in accordance with the rule, but behaves as though a different rule is in operation, and tests out the consequences. For example, Evelyn believed 'I must always help out others in need: If I don't they'll think badly of me and never speak to me again'. She practised with her neighbour: when she came round unexpectedly to talk about her problems, Evelyn told her she was busy but she was free for half an hour later on that day. Evelyn predicted that her friend would be very upset and angry and that Evelyn would feel awful if she were to do this. She predicted that she would experience chest pains if she was to be 'so rude'. She reported that her friend was, indeed, upset and angry and stormed off in tears. Evelyn did not, however, feel upset or experience chest pain: she felt angry that her friend had not understood that she was busy, and to her surprise her friend later came round to apologize for her behaviour and for 'taking Evelyn for granted'. As a result Evelyn felt closer to her friend.

The counsellor can encourage the client to begin to act in accordance with a new set of rules, and so test out the reality of the old assumptions and the advantages of the new assumptions. Other approaches to test assumptions include gaining information from other people to find out what their rules are; observing other's actions; and practising acting according to the new set of rules for a specified time and testing the consequences (Fennell, 1989).

It is extremely important for any experiments that the client and counsellor negotiate for them to be no-lose situations. Whatever the outcome of the experiment, the client must be able to learn something useful. Taking risks is, by definition, threatening to the client; therefore the client needs to be supported in the decision to try something new, with a good outcome whatever happens.

Working with core beliefs

There are important differences in the approaches for working with a client's assumptions and working with core beliefs or schema (Beck et al., 1990; Young, 1990; Young and Klosko, 1993). Assumptions are usually slightly easier to modify than are core beliefs, and therefore may be more amenable to shorter-term work. In contrast, counselling focusing on identifying and modifying a client's core beliefs may be far longer-term work, requiring much more emphasis on developing and maintaining a long-term therapeutic relationship (Safran and Segal, 1990; Young, 1990). The level at which it is necessary to work may vary according to the types of problem the client is dealing with. For example, working with clients with relatively short-term somatic symptoms, such as a relatively brief episode of health anxiety, irritable bowel symptoms or chest pains, may involve some work on the client's assumptions about the meaning of the symptoms or the meaning of the stresses underlying the symptoms. These clients may have relatively flexible assumptions, amenable to short-term counselling. In contrast, clients with long-term problems affecting many areas of their functioning are likely to have very firmly held core beliefs about themselves and their symptoms. They may be very unwilling to identify, let alone modify, the beliefs which have characterized much of their lives. Therefore, to work towards schema modification with these people is likely to involve much longer-term work.

Learning a new set of beliefs may be compared to learning to write with the other hand: if one is right handed, learning to write with the left hand takes time, patience and practice. Under stress, or when not thinking, one will automatically start to write with the right hand. So it is with our beliefs: they need to be consciously worked on until they feel more comfortable, natural and familiar. For example, Young and Klosko (1993) outline several steps for a client to change a core belief relating to vulnerability including the following:

- Try to understand the origins of your belief.
- Make a list of all the things that you are afraid of such as being ill, losing control, dangers.
- Enlist other people's help in facing up to your fears.
- Work out the probability of each feared event occurring.
- Write out what you will do in these situations on a card to carry with you as a reminder.
- Begin to tackle each of your fears in imagery.
- Tackle the fears in real life.
- Reward yourself for each step you take.

It can be helpful for the client to begin to learn to distinguish between 'old me and new me' or 'old plan versus new plan' (Persons, 1989), so giving the idea of developing a new set of strategies in place of the old. For example, for a client who believed themselves to be vulnerable, 'old me' would react to a headache with fear, going to bed and making an appointment with the doctor just in case it signalled the start of something serious; 'new me' might carry on regardless of the headache, deciding to ignore it until it went away, or ask what kinds of stresses might be causing the headache.

Keeping a diary or log, over several months, of evidence in favour of the new beliefs enables the client to see the consequences and advantages of the new beliefs and provides concrete evidence to counteract the old beliefs (Greenberger and Padesky, 1995). For example, a client who believes 'I am vulnerable' can be encouraged to write down, each day, instances which demonstrated strength and coping, such as examples of physical symptoms which were ignored and then disappeared, examples of taking risks or taking more exercise than usual, and so on. When the old belief is activated, the client then has evidence on hand to help contradict the belief and so begin to form a new set of beliefs.

Difficulties in modifying assumptions and beliefs

Working with a client's assumptions and beliefs may reveal vital key issues that become the focus of counselling. For example, certain psychosomatic problems such as irritable bowel syndrome or long-term somatic problems may be linked with childhood sexual abuse. Although in the long term it may be helpful and appropriate for the client to work through these problems, in the short term revealing significant background trauma may be extremely upsetting and disabling for the client who is, to some extent, being protected from these painful emotions by the symptoms. Some clients may not thank the counsellor, at least initially, for changing the problems from a set of painful somatic symptoms to far more painful emotions. The symptoms may for some time have served a useful function, protecting the client from the emotional consequences of abuse. A client may think 'I would rather have my terrible gut pains than even think about what happened as a child'. For some clients, therefore, the goal of counselling may be to respect the client's symptoms, and reframe them as useful to the client. As stressed throughout this book, the pace of counselling, and what is revealed or left unsaid, has to be left to the client.

Assumptions are often seen as very much part of the individual, and may be culturally reinforced. Therefore, other people may not like the changes in an individual. For example, Evelyn's assumptions lay in the areas of her needing to look after others at the expense of her own health, not allowing herself to say no to others' demands, and 'The only legitimate way to ask for help or have time for myself is to be ill'. As she identified her rules, and began to be more assertive about her own needs, she had to deal with her husband's concern: he assumed she must be feeling ill in order to allow herself time off. She had to deal with others' response to her saying no to their demands. At times she found it easier to go along with the 'old me' style of operating than to begin to look after herself better. At these times, the symptoms may become a warning sign that the old, unhelpful set of rules are in operation. The client can then make a choice as to whether to act in accordance with the old set of rules, which may in the short term be easier, despite giving rise to symptoms, or whether to try out the new set of rules.

In conclusion

Helping the client to identify and modify assumptions and beliefs which may underlie the somatic problems can help to reduce the client's vulnerability to developing future problems and can help the client to modify the meaning of somatic or psychological problems. The chapter has distinguished between working at the level of the client's unhelpful assumptions, which may be amenable to short-term counselling, and modifying core beliefs, which often involves longer-term therapy and a greater emphasis on the therapeutic relationship. Key skills and approaches in identifying and modifying assumptions include the use of questioning, imagery and metaphor, and encouraging the client to do experiments to test out a new set of rules. Identifying and modifying assumptions and beliefs can be the stage where the client may feel most vulnerable, and where the importance of a sound therapeutic relationship must be stressed. It is often the time when difficulties begin to emerge, as discussed in Chapter 7.

7

Difficulties and Problems in Counselling for Psychosomatic Problems

As stressed throughout the book, counselling clients with psycho-somatic problems may pose particular difficulties and issues for the counsellor, for the client and for the counselling relationship. These people also pose difficulties for the medical system, which is, as yet, far from well set up to deal with people with medically unexplained symptoms who have not found conventional medical treatments helpful, or where psychological factors are involved. This chapter looks in greater detail at some of these problems and suggests possible resolutions. Difficulties in the therapeutic relationship posed by working with this client group are described and suggestions are offered as to how to understand and work with these difficulties. The chapter discusses several key issues: managing anger towards the medical profession, particularly when the client and counsellor share similar feelings; setting limits on the client's behaviour, particularly seeking reassurance or when the client repeatedly consults other health professionals outside the counselling contract; working with clients who present with multiple symptoms or where, once one problem is resolved, another set of symptoms appear; working with clients who do not want to or cannot change; and suggestions for dealing with the situation when clients drop out of counselling. Finally, the chapter considers when counselling cannot help, and where a damage limitation exercise may be more appro-priate than any psychological intervention.

Difficulties and issues in the therapeutic relationship

> The therapeutic relationship: 'Two people, both with problems in living, who agree to work together to study those problems, with the hope that the counsellor has fewer problems than the patient. (Cited in Safran and Segal, 1990: 5)

Until recently, the therapeutic relationship received relatively little attention in cognitive therapy. In contrast to other forms of psycho-therapy, the task of cognitive therapy was seen to be to resolve the client's problems, as far as possible, using the tools of cognitive therapy rather than using the therapeutic relationship *per se*. A good relationship had to be in place in order to do the work, and was seen as necessary *but not sufficient alone* for therapeutic change (Beck et al., 1979). Although this 'necessary but not sufficient' view of the therapeutic relationship has been central to cognitive therapy, more attention is now being paid to the importance of the therapeutic relationship. Various studies looking at the relative contribution of non-specific, relationship factors versus technical factors in therapy indicate that relationship factors affect outcome in an interactive or additive way (DeRubeis and Feeley, 1990; Wright and Davis, 1994), a positive relationship making a significant contribution to the outcome of cognitive therapy (Burns and Nolen-Hoeksema, 1992; Persons, 1989; Persons and Burns, 1985). There is also more attention being paid to ways in which the therapeutic relationship itself can be used as an active ingredient in therapy (Beck et al., 1990; Jacobson, 1989; Safran, 1990; Safran and Segal, 1990; Young, 1990).

Cognitive therapy emphasizes the importance of developing a *collaborative relationship* and *collaborative empiricism* (Beck et al., 1979, 1985). In developing a good therapeutic collaboration, counsellors should be warm, open, empathic, concerned, respectful and non-judgemental. The process of developing such a collaborative relationship involves working with the client to set goals for counselling, determine priorities, maintain a therapeutic focus and structure, both within sessions and across counselling as a whole.

Defining difficulties in the therapeutic relationship
Difficulties in the therapeutic relationship can be broadly defined as anything to do with the relationship which means that the 'core conditions' of counselling are being compromised, or vanish altogether. Safran and Segal (1990) define therapeutic alliance 'ruptures' as any form of difficulty when the quality of the therapeutic alliance is strained or impaired. A rupture may be on a continuum from a simple misunderstanding during a session, to more chronic problems affecting the whole counselling. The cornerstone of cognitive counselling is the collaborative relationship: this, however, is not always easy to achieve, and one of the common relationship difficulties arises from problems with collaboration. Rather than both client and counsellor working together, in an open manner, to resolve the client's difficulties, the counsellor may become 'the expert' and start to offer directive advice; tasks may be set, not negotiated; the client may become 'over compliant' or 'non compliant', for example 'agreeing' with the counsellor on homework tasks and then not carrying them out. The counsellor may get the

feeling of being a 'bully', 'teacher' or 'political campaigner' in the sessions. The counsellor may lack empathy, or not be able to understand the client, or have extreme negative or positive feelings towards the client, causing difficulties in remaining an objective collaborator. Difficulties may express themselves as client 'resistance' (Newman, 1994), where the client may not collaborate or cooperate with counselling, or may 'go through the motions' of counselling without being fully engaged. The client may avoid looking at issues of importance previously agreed on, or avoid feeling or expressing any emotion, making the sessions dry and sterile. Alternatively, the client may express high levels of emotion towards the counsellor (Layden et al., 1993). 'Cognitive transference' describes the process where deeply held beliefs and well-ingrained patterns of behaviour are repeated in the therapeutic relationship and interfere with the collaborative relationship (Beck et al., 1990; Wright and Davis, 1994; Young, 1990).

Problems may also arise if the client and counsellor do not share the same conceptualization of the client's problems, so both are working to different agendas. For example, with clients who have somatic problems, it may be comparatively easy for the counsellor to arrive at a working conceptualization of the problem and the client may agree, in principle, with the model but not believe that it applies to them personally. These differences can cause relationship difficulties even before counselling commences.

Although, on paper, it is possible to define and describe difficulties in the therapeutic relationship, actual difficulties can be hard to describe in practice and may be missed. The therapeutic relationship involves engagement at the level of emotion and of interpersonal communication which may be non-verbal, and is therefore, at times, hard to describe. However, when difficulties are encountered, something almost intangible may occur: a vague feeling of discomfort, or behaviours that on the surface look straightforward but do not 'ring true', such as counsellor or client being persistently late for sessions, always armed with a 'good excuse'. Only when stepping back and trying to describe and analyse what is occurring, can the difficulties be understood and conceptualized.

Conceptualizing the client   Difficulties in the therapeutic relationship are very likely to mirror the client's psychological make-up, core beliefs and assumptions (Beck et al., 1990; Persons, 1989; Safran, 1990; Safran and Segal, 1990; Wright and Davis, 1994). Having a good conceptualization or formulation of the client, as described in Chapters 4 and 6, can predict possible difficulties in the therapeutic relationship. The therapeutic relationship is affected by the processes of schema maintenance described by Young (1990). In the therapeutic relationship, it is likely that clients will be 'testing out' the counsellor to check for a good 'fit' with their assumptions and beliefs, a process which the psychodynamic world describes as a 'transference test'. For example, the belief that 'I'm boring' may lead the client to speak or behave in a flat, boring manner, or selectively attend to any tiny cues that the counsellor is finding them boring.

Problems in the relationship can be linked to the client's fundamental beliefs about interpersonal relationships or specific helping relationships. For example, people who have a strong need for advice, information and reassurance about their health will have evolved specific, and possibly subtle, behaviours to get reassurance. The counsellor may link in with this and become a 'friendly expert', agreeing with the client how difficult it is to squeeze information out of doctors. If, conversely, the client believes that all medical people are to be disbelieved, often based on personal experience of mis-information from or misunderstandings with the medical profession, then the client may well treat the counsellor with suspicion. The client may apparently go along with the process of counselling but be on the lookout for clues that the counselling is not working or that the counsellor has got it wrong. Addressing the client's suspicions is extremely important in beginning to restore the therapeutic relationship.

The client's assumptions and beliefs about relationships may force the counsellor into a 'damned if I do, damned if I don't' situation (Layden et al., 1993). This feeling is characteristic of working with clients where their experiences and resulting schema mean that whatever others do, it can be misconstrued in a negative way, resulting in a 'no win' situation in close relationships. As a response, the counsellor can also react in a black and white way: either responding to the client's outbursts and irrational demands by eagerness to end counselling and discharge the client, labelling them as 'impossible to help'; or, at the other extreme, the counsellor may become a rescuer, going to unusual extremes to help the client or offer the client unrealistic assurances about the counsellor's ability to help, inevitably leading the client to feel disillusioned or betrayed. The therapeutic relationship may 'ping pong' back and forward between the two extremes of over distance and over involvement, mirroring the client's schema and problems. The following example illustrates the effects of the client's beliefs on the therapeutic relationship.

'Ian' believed that 'no one is to be trusted', compensated by an assumption that 'if I search long and hard enough, I'll be able to find the one person who can help me with my problems'. He had spent years consulting doctors, in several different countries, for help with persistent physical symptoms; during this time he had also collected numerous examples of medical incompetence, as his frequent tests inevitably had their side effects. From the start of counselling, I would find myself subtly manoeuvred into situations where I did not know the answers, which proved his point. I became, inevitably, frustrated and irritated with him, and found myself feeling completely incompetent. I wanted to discharge him quickly, thereby confirming his beliefs that no one could help him.

Conceptualizing the counsellor   Counsellors are only too human. We have our own 'blind spots and particular areas of sensitivity' which inevitably interact with the client's problems (Layden et al., 1993). Our schema, assumptions and experiences lead us to act, react and feel in certain ways in counselling. Therefore, understanding difficulties in the therapeutic relationship must involve understanding the contribution of the counsellor as well as that of the client.

The classic psychoanalytical view maintains that 'countertransference' is the counsellor's *unconscious* reaction to the client's transference, and has its base in the counsellor's unresolved neurotic conflicts. In cognitive therapy, countertransference is viewed as a valuable means of gaining a deeper understanding of the therapeutic process; it represents the totality of the counsellor's responses to the client, including thoughts, schemas, emotions, actions and intentions (Layden et al., 1993). Counsellors' feelings and reactions are used 'in the service of therapy rather than allowing them to become obstacles in therapy' (Safran and Segal, 1990: 41).

It is helpful if the counsellor is aware of her or his own rules, assumptions and schema which may interfere with the ability to either identify or discuss difficulties in the therapeutic relationship. Assumptions such as 'it is wrong to disagree with or feel attracted to or be angry with my clients', 'I should not dislike my client', or 'I must cure the patient', are likely to interfere with the therapeutic relationship: if the counsellor has particular feelings or thoughts that contravene these rules, then they may be ignored or put back on to the client, rather than actively used in counselling. The counsellor may feel insecure about their level of medical knowledge about the client's particular problems. The counsellor may have thoughts such as 'I must be shown to know something about this problem' leading the counsellor to become 'the expert', over-professional and knowledgeable, to the detriment of collaboration. Safran and Segal (1990) stress that the counsellor needs to have a sufficiently flexible, and accepting, self-concept to be able to acknowledge and accept her or his own feelings in the therapeutic interaction.

Environmental factors   Various factors external to the client and counsellor may cause difficulties in the therapeutic relationship (Wright and Davis, 1994). These include the type or length of counselling; the situation, such as hospital versus primary-care-based counselling; pressures to 'cure' people in a fixed length of time; social or cultural factors; financial issues; or effects of the client's social circumstances. Difficulties in the therapeutic relationship may reflect a mismatch between the client's needs and the counsellor's style or mode of counselling. The high level of structure, questioning, or empirical approach suggested in cognitive counselling may not suit some clients, being so incompatible with their beliefs and assumptions as to make developing a therapeutic relationship extremely difficult. Alternatively, a less structured form of counselling, focusing on the therapeutic relationship, may be very threatening and difficult for some clients.

Working on difficulties in the therapeutic relationship
Conceptualizing and working with difficulties in the therapeutic relationship assumes that these difficulties are a product of the same kind of patterns of thinking, unhelpful assumptions or schema as are any other difficulties, particularly interpersonal difficulties. Therefore, such problems can be identified, understood and worked with in the same way in cognitive counselling as are the client's presenting problems. The extra factor is that the counsellor's own patterns of thinking, unhelpful assumptions or schema are also relevant, and need to be conceptualized and worked with. A number of stages are involved in working with difficulties in the therapeutic relationship: assessment and weaving the issues into the conceptualization, then collaboratively sharing and working on the issues with the client. As discussed in Chapter 3, the value and importance of supervision when identifying and working with difficulties in the counselling process must be stressed: because of the nature of the therapeutic relationship, it is often difficult even to spot that there are potential or actual pitfalls without supervision from others.

Assessment and conceptualization   The first step to working with difficulties in the therapeutic relationship is to identify and assess what is going on (Safran and Segal, 1990; Newman, 1994). Some problems are immediately obvious, for example if the client and counsellor end up 'arguing', or the counsellor feels strongly negative towards the client. However, it can also be very difficult to identify problems or difficulties at the time, since we are by definition a participant in the relationship with the client, and our behaviour will inevitably be affected by the encounter. Both counsellor and client are likely to 'pull' from each other behaviours or emotional responses that will maintain their schema. Difficulties can therefore be identified when reflected on after a counselling session, using counselling tapes, discussion with colleagues and supervision. The key to assessing difficulties is initially to become an objective observer of, rather than a participant in, the difficulties.

Safran and Segal (1990) describe means of identifying 'rupture markers' when the therapeutic relationship becomes strained or impaired. The first step is to become a 'participant observer', using 'decentering' – the process of stepping outside one's immediate experience and thereby not only observing the experience but also changing the nature of the experience itself. In psychoanalytic therapy, the process is called developing an 'observing ego' or developing the 'observing self'. Rather than simply being part of and reacting to an encounter, or being 'hooked' in the interaction, such as may happen during conversation outside of counselling, the counsellor is also aware of being a participant in the encounter. The counsellor then 'unhooks' from the interaction to avoid becoming so engaged in the interaction that clients' schema are, yet again, confirmed (Kiesler, 1988).

> Ian, for example, was both wanting help from the counsellor and wanting to prove that the counsellor could not help him. During the 'hooked' stage of counselling, the client's behaviour forces the counsellor into a narrow and restricted range of responses: to Ian's questions about his symptoms, the counsellor can only respond by desperately trying to be 'the expert' and answer all his questions. In the unhooked stage, the first task is to notice, attend to and try and label what is being pulled from the counsellor by the client. The second task involves 'unhooking' and discontinuing with the usual responses, and discussing what is going on, such as reflecting 'I feel like I'm being tested to see how much I know: I wonder what went through your mind just before you said x . . . what you are feeling right now?' By using this process, gaining supervision and dealing with my own negative reactions, Ian continued counselling and began to look at his mistrust: neither client nor counsellor gave up on the other.

Much of interpersonal communication takes place at a non-verbal level, making it difficult, at times, to define why the counsellor is reacting in a certain way. The counsellor's bodily reactions, images or metaphors can provide useful clues to the conceptualization.

When working with clients with somatic problems, the counsellor may experience some of the client's symptoms or notice changes in her or his own bodily state: my own experience of flatulence, stomach pains and altered bowel activity when working with a group of clients with bowel symptoms is testimony to this phenomenon! The counsellor's images about themselves or about the client can provide important clues as to relationship issues and the client's conceptualization. Feeling like a 'wise owl' or other symbol of wisdom may identify the client's need for reassurance. If, conversely, the client believes that all medics are to be disbelieved, then the client may well treat the counsellor with suspicion: the counsellor may feel like trying exceptionally hard, and against all odds, to 'sell' the client the model of counselling, and may feel like an 'estate agent'.

Newman (1994) suggests a number of questions that the counsellor can use to assess difficulties. Although it is suggested that the counsellor ask these questions about the client, it is also useful for the counsellor to assess their role in the difficulties:

- What is the function of the client's behaviour? What does the client fear will happen if the difficulties were not there? For example, being angry with the counsellor may protect the client from other, more painful feelings.
- How do the problems fit with the longitudinal or developmental conceptualization? When and under what circumstances has the client been similarly affected in the past?
- What counsellor or client beliefs are feeding the current situation? How might the client or counsellor be characteristically misunderstanding or misinterpreting the other or the situation, i.e. what schema maintenance behaviours are in operation?
- Do the counsellor or client lack certain skills which make it difficult to collaborate with counselling or resolve the present difficulties? For example, either client or counsellor may have problems with assertiveness which are causing difficulties.
- Are there environmental factors influencing the counselling? For example, the client's partner may fear change, and so may actively block the client's 'homework' assignments.
- Does the conceptualization need revision? For example, a client who says 'you don't understand', may be right because the counsellor may be overlooking important points because they do not fit with the counsellor's conceptualization.

Collaboration Once difficulties are identified and assessed, counsellor and client work together to conceptualize and deal with the difficulties. This process must be guided by the conceptualization, and is both an extremely valuable and potentially 'dangerous' stage of counselling. Interventions focusing on the relationship can be very threatening to clients who have had no experience of being able to discuss or resolve relationship difficulties. It can be useful to use 'here and now' examples within the session to explore difficulties and identify the client's thoughts and feelings at times of alliance ruptures. The counsellor can ask the client: 'when I said x, it looked as though it was uncomfortable: what went through your mind just then?' or 'When I said x, you seemed to close off – was there something about it that was familiar . . . have you felt like this before . . . did it remind you of something?'

When giving any kind of feedback to clients about what is going on in the relationship, counsellors must acknowledge their own contribution to the experience, and not blame or pathologize the client. Rather than saying, 'I feel like you are . . .' the counsellor can offer their own feelings: 'I feel like I am giving you a lecture at the moment, and am not sure why this is', or 'I feel quite puzzled when you tell me you are sad but laugh at the same time'. If the counsellor is able to be 'real' and admit to mistakes or uncertainties, this can be both a powerful model and a means of challenging assumptions or schema within sessions. Clients with somatic problems may have had repeated experiences of their problems being seen as 'their fault' rather than because of the limitations of medicine; being able to say 'I don't know', 'I feel like I should have all the answers about your physical problems, and it is difficult not to know', can begin to challenge beliefs about 'someone, out there, has the answers to my difficulties'.

Dealing with the counsellor's difficulties   Layden et al. (1993) describe some of the characteristics required of counsellors to enable them to work with difficulties in the therapeutic relationship. The counsellor needs to be a 'real person', who acts in a consistently positive, supportive manner, maintaining a firm grounding in reality, an even temperament, and being willing to address difficulties in the therapeutic relationship as they occur. The counsellor must be secure enough to admit to mistakes, and have non-judgemental self aware-ness. No doubt we all, at times, fall short of these requirements, and difficulties in the therapeutic relationship may arise from the coun-sellor's particular experience and psychology. Clients with somatic problems may remind of us of our own vulnerabilities or periods of ill health, or the ways in which we all face uncertainties about our health. It can be helpful for the counsellor to monitor their thoughts about the client or the counselling process, using a diary of thoughts (see Table 5.3), monitoring any feelings about the client and associated thoughts. Thought diaries and downward arrow techniques can also help the counsellor to identify assumptions and beliefs that may underlie reactions to the client (Persons, 1989). Counselling tapes can be very useful to identify negative thoughts or other reactions to clients (Wright and Davis, 1994). Other techniques include cognitive rehearsal and role play in supervision to anticipate and work with difficulties in sessions. Weaving the issues into the conceptualization is a powerful means of dealing with the counsellor's own negative reactions to the client.

Difficulties in empathizing with the client A common difficulty in the therapeutic relationship can be difficulty in empathizing with the client. The sessions may shift from seeming 'alive', with a sense of counsellor and client working together in an active way, to a 'dead' feeling, where both participants are 'going through the motions' of counselling in the absence of therapeutic change. There may be various reasons for this. The counsellor may have a negative reaction to the client, as discussed above. Some clients with somatic problems, who are not fully engaged with counselling, may go through the counselling with the covert agenda of demonstrating to the counsellor that the counselling is not effective, so giving more credence to their view that their problems are 'real' and 'physical': 'I did just what you told me to and it did not work'. The counsellor may feel frustration with or disbelief of the client, or disparaged by the client. It is important for the counsellor to be able to step back from these reactions, think about what is going on, and try and understand in terms of the client's conceptualization. It can be helpful for the counsellor to ask him or herself 'If I had this background and set of beliefs, how would I be feeling or thinking in response to x.'

Managing anger towards the medical profession

Many clients will be angry towards doctors and towards previous treatments or what they see as inadequate or unhelpful treatments. Clients often express intense anger towards the counsellor. The client may want the counsellor to help to make a complaint against a doctor; alternatively the client may see the counsellor as 'on the side' of the medics. Being able to work with this anger without either dismissing or colluding with it is a key skill in counselling. How this anger is dealt with can have an important effect on the outcome of counselling.

It is particularly important for the counsellor to be able to disentangle what is going on for the client from the counsellor's own view about the medical profession or medical treatments. The counsellor may agree, from the client's story, that the client has had a 'raw deal' but it may be unhelpful to blame others in a simplistic way without checking the possible contribution of the client. For example, a client may have extremely unrealistic expectations about what medicine can offer; the client may repeatedly ignore the doctor's suggestions and yet repeatedly ask for advice; the client may demand further consultations for test results which take some time to complete; the doctor may have told the client several times that the tests were negative, and may find it difficult to manage the client's constant disbelief. When faced with a client's anger towards others, it is important for the counsellor to be able to clarify what really happened. The counsellor can then gently confront the client's behaviour, exploring what feelings were motivating the client, and whether the client has realistic expectations of the doctor's powers (Murphy, 1993). The client may be asking for help in a way that means that the client is least likely to get help. It is important to acknowledge the client's feelings without necessarily agreeing with the basis for them. On hearing some client's stories, it is easy to feel that justice has not been done; however, gaining the 'other side of the story' is sometimes illuminating.

Setting limits and containment

Setting limits means deciding on what is acceptable within the counselling setting. It involves limits on session times, numbers and what is acceptable within sessions. Some clients may repeatedly telephone or turn up at the counsellor's workplace when the symptoms are bad, needing immediate help. Setting limits on such help-seeking behaviour is very important to the therapeutic relationship and may involve helping the client to understand feelings of abandonment or discomfort if help is not immediately available. Setting limits means the counsellor does not collude or take sides with the client, but will help the client understand his or her feelings about the situation and what it may be realistic to try and do. Some clients may agree with the counsellor not to consult others for help during the process of counselling, but may go against this, and repeatedly return to the doctor, seek private medical consultations or consult alternative practitioners. The counselling may begin to take the form of one professional opinion being played against another. It is helpful for the client and counsellor to negotiate how much and under what circumstances the client uses other forms of help during counselling: clearly some consultations are entirely appropriate. The client may, however, be using others to gain reassurance which may or may not be helpful. This must be addressed during counselling. Alternatively, rather than seeing the doctor in a panic about new symptoms, it may be that the client needs more reassurance and support from the doctor than the client is currently getting. It would therefore be more appropriate to negotiate regular sessions with the general practitioner, such as a once-monthly appointment regardless of how the client is feeling, which may in the long term reduce the need for panic consultations.

The counsellor is containing the client by tolerating the client's anger, hostility or other emotions, while remaining empathic and emotionally available to the client. The counsellor must continue to try and understand the client's behaviour and feelings, and communicate this understanding to the client. It is particularly important with this client group to try and stay with the difficulties: many may have had experiences of rejection from others who perceive them as too demanding or impossible, or from doctors who become frustrated by the patient never believing medical opinions or taking medical advice despite repeatedly asking for help.

Clients with multiple symptoms

At least at the beginning of counselling, the focus is often on one symptom, broadening out to look at other problems and underlying psychological mechanisms. Clients with more severe forms of psychosomatic problems and a general tendency to somatize any distress may have many symptoms which are rather vaguely defined. The meaning given to specific symptoms may also be vague, making it more difficult to target and work with a client's problems. If counselling begins by focusing on one symptom, this may reduce only to find another medically unexplained symptom emerging. Some clients may report various symptoms apparently travelling the course of their bodies. Although the counsellor may be tempted to work on the symptoms as they emerge, and often the pull from the client is to become involved with each symptom, it is more helpful to stand back and see the underlying processes, identifying and working with the underlying assumptions and schema. Key themes may be 'Any symptom must mean something serious'; 'I must always pay attention to my body: otherwise I may miss something'; or 'I am the sort of person who is vulnerable to illnesses'. However, just because an individual is anxious about their health or has a tendency to experience somatic symptoms when under stress, does not mean they are immune to diseases. As discussed in Chapter 3, the client and counsellor have to balance the psychological needs of the client with the need to take good care of themselves and consult doctors or other health carers when it is appropriate.

Clients who do not want to or cannot change

However hard the counsellor or client may work in counselling, however good the therapeutic relationship and the conceptualization of the client, there may be powerful reasons against a client changing. If the client is pursuing a compensation claim, or is seeking retirement on medical grounds, then the client may be going through the process of counselling with the covert agenda of proving how ill they are, and disproving the role of psychological factors. In this case, counselling is likely to be completely ineffective.

Some clients may gain a great deal from their symptoms. Although the notion of 'secondary gain' is often used in a pejorative manner, it may be valuable to look at the function of symptoms and what the client may lose by getting better. Illness can be a valuable coping strategy rather than an unwanted set of symptoms. For example, migraines may be the only way that an individual is able to get time alone in an otherwise over-filled life. Being ill is socially endorsed and an acceptable reason for slowing down or having a rest. Although some workplaces offer compassionate leave or 'mental health days', it is often the case that the only way the individual can begin to look after her or himself is to be ill. Other people may benefit from the client's illness: for example, the balance of a long-term marriage may depend on the husband being the weaker, ill party and the wife looking after him, which would lead to relationship problems should the husband get better. Change may involve considerable costs to the client, both financial and emotional. A client who is off work may lose sickness or disability benefits, or going back to work would force the client to face up to the need to change an unsatisfactory career. For example, a client who was coping with chronic arm pains diagnosed as tenosynovitis, was able to see that the pains had helped her to leave a job which she disliked, which she felt she had to 'hold on to' at all costs.

The counselling can both explore the individual's beliefs which may maintain problems and look at the symptoms in the wider social context. Part of counselling may involve re-framing the symptoms as useful to the client and therefore less of a problem.

People who drop out of counselling

It is not uncommon for clients with somatic problems to drop out of counselling, often at an early stage. Some of the guidelines offered in

Chapter 3 may help to engage clients in counselling and so reduce the likelihood of the client ending counselling prematurely (Guthrie, 1995). Should the individual drop out of counselling, it may be appropriate to contact the client and if possible discuss the reasons for not wanting to continue counselling. The conceptualization may need to be reviewed and revised: it may reflect the counsellor's understanding of the client's problems but not the client's under-standing. There may be misunderstandings about the role of counselling that need to be clarified, or significant others, such as a partner or family members, may be discouraging the client from attending. It may be appropriate to offer another session in which these others can discuss their reservations.

However, as discussed throughout this book, a number of clients will not feel that counselling is appropriate or has anything to offer, and these feelings must be respected. Sometimes, working with the general practitioner or the referring doctor to help them better manage and help the client may be more appropriate than trying to continue to see a reluctant client.

When counselling cannot help

Although the counsellor may genuinely want to work with and try and help individuals with psychosomatic problems, in some cases even beginning counselling may be counterproductive. People with severe, long-term problems characterizing somatization disorder may be particularly difficult to help. These people may have life-long problems in functioning, associated with a number of symp-toms which change at different times. An experience of failure in counselling may lead the client to reject completely the role of psychological factors and to add psychological therapists to their list of people who are unable to help them. However, these individuals may be at risk of iatrogenic problems, such as the risks associated with repeated tests or medical investigations or long-term use of prescribed and over-the-counter medications. 'Damage limitation' may be a more realistic goal than cure, aiming to help the client to reduce their use of medical investigations or treatments when not necessary, or helping the doctor to set limits on the amount of unnecessary tests the client receives. Joint sessions between the client, counsellor and general practitioner can be helpful. The counsellor can then help the general practitioner develop goals and guidelines for managing the client. It may be appropriate for the doctor, or counsellor, to offer regular follow-up appointments to offer the client support and help the client reduce or limit their use of other medical services when not medically indicated.

One of the strongest predictors of a good outcome to psychological therapies is if the client is able to acknowledge and work with psychological distress. For clients who are not psychologically distressed or who are unwilling or unable to acknowledge their feelings, approaches that do not focus on emotions and feelings may be more helpful (Guthrie, 1995). For these people, more 'physical-based' approaches may be appropriate: for example, hypnotherapy can be effective in reducing symptoms in people with irritable bowel syndrome who do not report psychological distress (Harvey et al., 1987; Whorwell et al., 1984). Other alternative therapies may be helpful in managing the client's symptoms and offering psychological support, while not necessarily working directly on psychological problems.

Some individuals, in a small minority, may have extremely strong beliefs about their health which may be so strong as to be delusional. Helping these people requires specialist psychiatric treatment. Some people, again in a small minority, may have 'factitious' or manufactured problems, such as deliberately causing bowel symptoms, by overdosing with laxatives or other medications, and then denying that they are harming themselves. These people, again, may well need specialist help from psychiatry as opposed to counselling. It is extremely important for counsellors to know and recognize the limits of what they can offer and when a psychiatric opinion is needed.

A note of caution

There may be very occasional cases in a counsellor's history where the client and counsellor work well together, develop a good conceptualization of the client's problems, work on the presenting problems and underlying issues in a collaborative way, enable the client to cope with the symptoms, and minimize all reassurance seeking and 'inappropriate' medical consultations. Despite all the predictors of a good outcome being in place, the client continues to experience symptoms. Medical practitioners and the tools of their trade are fallible and mistakes in diagnosis do occur. Psychological difficulties do not make a client immune to physical problems and may even predispose the individual to developing illnesses or diseases. If the client does not improve, it may for some people be appropriate for the client to seek further medical advice or tests. This involves a careful balance between the client's medical needs and the psychological needs, for example using medical practitioners for repeated reassurance. It may be more difficult for the client to gain medical investigations if the medical practitioners believe that receiving psychological therapy means that the symptoms must be 'psychological'. The stage of counselling and moving back to further medical investigations needs to be carefully and sensitively negotiated with all concerned.

In conclusion

This chapter has considered some of the difficulties and issues that arise when working with clients with psychosomatic problems. The difficulties are not unique to this client group and will have been encountered in many instances in counselling. For further reading on these issues, the reader is referred to Dryden (1989a, 1989b) and Mearns and Dryden (1990). One of the key ways of dealing with difficulties is to formulate or conceptualize the difficulties in terms of both client and counsellor, considering the interaction between the two. Working with this client group requires flexibility on the part of the counsellor, being able to adapt the counselling approach according to the needs of the client. Gaining regular supervision is essential in order to negotiate some of the minefields described in this chapter. When clients disparage us and our methods, drop out of counselling, complain that, despite our best efforts we are not taking them seriously, or make formal complaints against us, having a supervisor on hand to help pick up the pieces and restore ourselves as well as the therapeutic relationship, is essential.

8

Ending Counselling and Long-term Coping

> Termination is more than an act signifying the end of therapy; it is an integral part of the process of therapy and, if properly understood and managed, may be an important factor in the instigation of change. (Yalom, 1975: 365)

Although ending counselling follows general principles discussed by Ward (1989) there are some issues in ending counselling that may be of particular relevance to counselling clients with psychosomatic problems. Addressing the ending of counselling is, at times, inadequately handled (Ward, 1989). One way of understanding the end of counselling is to conceptualize it as a process or stage rather than a sudden cessation of activity, which needs to be given an appropriate amount of time and attention. For a number of reasons, it is particularly important to address the ending of counselling for clients with psychosomatic problems. If the ending is handled inappropriately, the individual may not seek further psychological help when needed, and may turn again, inappropriately, to medical practitioners. If the development of somatic symptoms is related to emotional and relationship issues, the ending of counselling may re-evoke feelings of loss and rejection which need to be addressed before the ending of the counselling relationship. The client may have long-term experiences of somatic symptoms enabling the client to remain in relationships: this may be repeated in the counselling relationship, so that the potential loss of the counsellor re-evokes the client's need for the symptoms. The client may face setbacks or relapses in future, which need to be planned for before counselling ends. When to offer follow-up and long-term support needs to be discussed and decided during the end stages of counselling.

Having a good conceptualization or formulation of the client's beliefs and assumptions is invaluable in predicting and working with difficulties in ending counselling. For example, schema concerned with dependency on others, beliefs that the client is unable to cope alone, beliefs that the only way of keeping another person in a relationship is to be ill, are likely to be activated during the ending of counselling, particularly if the client and counsellor have formed a good therapeutic relationship. For other clients, where counselling has been less helpful, beliefs may be activated and strengthened such as 'no one can help me'.

Ending counselling may involve three stages (Ward, 1989). The first stage involves assessing the client's readiness for the end of counselling. The second stage involves addressing and resolving remaining issues and bringing about appropriate closure of the relationship between client and counsellor. The third stage enables the client to consolidate what has been gained and learned during counselling and to carry on using these gains after counselling has ended. The extent to which each of these three stages is emphasized depends on the individual client and the counselling situation.

Assessing when to end counselling

The usual criteria for when to stop counselling are when the client feels better about the presenting problems and is acting differently in life, or at least working in that direction. The client's goals for counselling and the extent to which they have been met needs to be the main factor guiding the end of counselling. However, it is important that these goals are realistic. Counselling is not likely to resolve all problems, remove all symptoms or result in a 'complete cure'. It is often the case that clients who present with somatic concerns may well still experience the symptoms that led them to seek help in the first place. The aim is for the client to be less anxious about the problems, less limited by the symptoms, less likely to make repeated unhelpful medical consultations and risk the consequent iatrogenic problems, and to be focusing more on other problems or difficulties that need to be addressed, for example working through relationship issues or dealing with stress. It is also not realistic for the client to expect never to feel anxious, low, upset or angry again. An important goal of counselling is to be able to normalize distress. This may be particularly important for clients who have not been able to express or experience emotional distress, who may be feeling significantly more emotionally fluid since starting counselling, perhaps feeling and expressing emotions in a way which was previously uncharacteristic of the individual.

David had very mixed feelings about ending counselling. Although some of his initial goals had been to get rid of his symptoms, he was surprised at the results of counselling. He was continuing to experience symptoms, but they posed far less of a problem to him. He was able to make the links between the various stresses in his life and the symptoms and realized that his fears about losing control of his bowels were exaggerated. He had begun to look at his assumptions about having to cope, be in control and keep his feelings to himself, and had begun to talk about the problems in his relationship. He reported in some ways feeling worse: he began to feel sad about his plight and about the years he had missed out on close relationships while having to keep his feelings to himself. He was feeling angry, too – an emotion that was alien to him. Part of him wanted to end counselling and retreat back into himself; part of him wanted to continue the journey he had started and was concerned about ending counselling. We spent some time discussing the ending stages of counselling: how he could use his feelings rather than return to bottling them up; how his bowel symptoms may prove a useful indicator of his emotional state rather than a set of problems to get rid of; and how he could gain support and help from other people in his life.

The number of counselling sessions, and therefore the end of counselling, may well be fixed by practical constraints caused by factors external to the client and counsellor. Particularly when working in the health service, the number of counselling sessions it is possible to offer a client is limited, often to 10 sessions for short-term work or 20 sessions for longer-term work. Working within a limited number of sessions helps the counselling maintain a structure and focus, helps to make the best use of the available time, and may give the client the important message that the problems are manageable and solutions can be found in a relatively brief period of time. Limits on counselling may also mean that important issues can only be touched upon and not fully addressed. Whatever the length of counselling, the limit is discussed and negotiated during the first session.

One way of beginning the end of counselling is to begin to increase the time between sessions. The counsellor and client may meet weekly during the initial stages of counselling, but may then spread out the sessions to every two or three weeks. This enables the client to have more time between sessions in which to practise and consolidate gains made during counselling, and also allows any potential difficulties to arise before counselling has ended.

Dealing with unresolved issues and ending the therapeutic relationship

During the final stages of counselling, the client may identify issues that have not been resolved during counselling. Although the focus of the counselling may have been on dealing with physical problems, the client may want to continue to work on social or psychological problems revealed during counselling. The client and counsellor can discuss how best to deal with these issues. It may be possible to negotiate a number of additional sessions; it may be more appropriate to look for other sources of help such as relationship counselling. Some clients may bring important issues to the last session, with the flavour of a 'parting shot', leaving the counsellor puzzled, frustrated or annoyed, which may mean the counselling ends with an unfinished feeling. It may be that these issues are too difficult or threatening for the client to work with them; they may be brought up as a way of continuing the therapeutic relationship. It is important to try and discuss what has happened and offer some understanding in terms of the client's conceptualization.

The end of the counselling relationship may evoke a variety of feelings including loss, grief or abandonment. Addressing and discussing these feelings is an important part of the stage of ending counselling. The client can be encouraged to look at any similarities between ending counselling and other endings. The client may be invited to think about how they usually handle saying goodbye, and whether the client wishes to try out a different, more satisfactory way of ending the relationship.

The counsellor also can look at their feelings at ending counselling. If the counsellor has found the client particularly difficult to work with, or counselling has not been particularly helpful, they may feel a sense of disappointment at not being able to help or relief at finishing with the client. Alternatively, sometimes it is difficult for us to end counselling at the point at which the client is improving or becoming more emotionally accessible and, therefore, more rewarding to work with. These feelings are often best dealt with during supervision.

Preparing for the future: long-term coping

The final stages of counselling are focused on helping the client to prepare for coping in the future, once counselling has ended. It is very valuable to review with the client what has been learned during counselling. It is not unusual for clients to experience setbacks during or after counselling. Although setbacks can be difficult to deal with, and the client may think 'I have gone back to square one', setbacks can be conceptualized as helpful to the client, giving the opportunity to identify and work on difficulties. The client can be encouraged to think about how to deal with setbacks, and not necessarily regard them as evidence of relapse. However, should the client relapse, how to deal with this and where to seek help, if

- What have you learned?
- What has been useful to you?
- How can you build on what you have learned? Describe a 'plan for action'.
- What will make it difficult for you to put this plan for action into practice?
- How will you deal with these difficulties?
- What might lead to a setback for you? For example, stresses, life problems, relationships, etc.
- If you do have a setback, what will you do about it?

Figure 8.1   *Counselling blueprint*

appropriate, can be discussed. The client can be invited to write a 'blueprint' for the end of counselling, to take away as a reminder of what was learned during counselling. Working on a blueprint involves at least two sessions for the client to think about the questions and work through them with the counsellor. An example of the kinds of questions to include on a blueprint is given in Figure 8.1.

Towards the end of counselling, the counsellor can act as 'devil's advocate' for the client: the client can put forward the arguments in favour of ending counselling and how to cope in future, and the counsellor can attempt to challenge these, to help the client clarify possible issues in ending counselling.

The client can be encouraged to carry on working on the issues identified during counselling after counselling has ended. An important goal is for the client to become his or her own therapist, or be able to use informal support networks rather than automatically relying on professional help.

Offering follow-up sessions
Many counsellors will routinely offer clients a follow-up session after counselling has ended in which to review progress and work on difficulties. Offering follow-up sessions may be valuable; however, continuing contact with the counsellor may be a means of the client gaining continuing and perhaps inappropriate or unhelpful reassurance. Follow-up sessions may be a way of client or counsellor avoiding saying goodbye and dealing with the resulting feelings of loss. It is important for the client and counsellor to be aware of the hazards as well as potential benefits of offering follow-up sessions.

At the end of counselling, Evelyn felt that many of her goals had been met. She noticed chest pains only occasionally and could clearly link these with being 'uptight'. Her problems made sense to her in terms of her long-term belief in being responsible for everyone else's well-being and she had made big steps in getting her own needs met and standing up for herself. Her family were initially unhappy about the changes in Evelyn, but were beginning to accept that she was going to do things differently from now on. Although her symptoms and medical tests had been frightening and difficult for her, she felt that the experience had been useful in the long run. She felt ready to end, but a little nervous about coping in future on her own. She arranged a follow-up session three months after the end of counselling 'just in case'. When the time came, Evelyn cancelled the appointment, feeling that she was happy to carry on without me.

References

American Psychiatric Association (1994). *Diagnostic and Statistical Manual of Mental Disorders. DSM-IV*. Washington DC: American Psychiatric Association.

Barsky, A.J. and Klerman, G.L. (1983). Overview: hypochondriasis, bodily complaints and somatic styles. *American Journal of Psychiatry*, 140: 273–81.

Barsky, A.J., Geringer, E. and Wool, C.A. (1988). A cognitive-educational treatment for hypochondriasis. *General Hospital Psychiatry*, 10: 322–7.

Barsky, A.J.M., Wool, C., Barnett, M.C. and Cleary, P.D. (1994). Histories of childhood trauma in adult hypochondriacal patients. *American Journal of Psychiatry*, 151 (3): 397–401.

Bass, C. (1990). *Somatization: Physical Symptoms and Psychological Illness*. Oxford: Blackwell Scientific Publications.

Bass, C. and Benjamin, S. (1993). The management of chronic somatisation. *British Journal of Psychiatry*, 162: 472–80.

Bass, C. and Murphy, M. (1995). Somatoform and personality disorders: Syndromal comorbidity and overlapping developmental pathways. *Journal of Psychosomatic Research*, 39 (4): 403–27.

Bass, C., Wade, C., Hand, D. and Jackson, G. (1983). Patients with angina with normal and near normal coronary arteries: clinical and psychosocial state 12 months after angiography. *British Medical Journal*, 287: 1505–8.

Bass, C., Chambers, J.B. and Gardner, W.N. (1991). Hyperventilation provocation in patients with chest pain and normal coronary arteries. *Journal of Psychosomatic Research*, 35: 83–9.

Beck, A.T. (1976). *Cognitive Therapy and the Emotional Disorders*. New York: International Universities Press.

Beck, A.T., Rush, A.J., Shaw, B.F. and Emery, G. (1979). *Cognitive Therapy of Depression*. New York: Guildford Press.

Beck, A.T., Emery, G. and Greenberg, R.L. (1985). *Anxiety Disorders and Phobias. A Cognitive Perspective*. New York: Basic Books.

Beck, A.T., Freeman, A. and Associates (1990). *Cognitive Therapy of Personality Disorders*. New York: Guildford Press.

Benjamin, S. (1989). Psychological treatment of chronic pain: a selective review. *Journal of Psychosomatic Research*, 33: 121–31.

Benjamin, S., Mawer, J. and Lennon, S. (1992). The knowledge and beliefs of family care givers about chronic pain patients. *Journal of Psychosomatic Research*, 36: 211–17.

Bhatt, A., Tomenson, B. and Benjamin, S. (1989). Transcultural patterns of somatisation in primary care: a preliminary report. *Journal of Psychosomatic Research*, 33 (6): 671–80.

Blackburn, I.M. and Davidson, K. (1990). *Cognitive Therapy for Depression and Anxiety*. Oxford: Blackwell Scientific Publications.

Blake, F., Gask, D. and Salkovskis, P. (1985). Psychological aspects of premenstrual syndrome: developing a cognitive approach. In R. Mayou, C. Bass and M. Sharpe (eds). *Treatment of Functional Somatic Symptoms.* Oxford: Oxford University Press. pp. 271–84.

Blanchard, E.B., Schwartz, S.P., Suls, J.M., Gerardi, M.A., Scharff, L., Greene, B., Taylor, A.E., Berreman, C. and Malamood, H.S. (1992). Two controlled evaluations of multi-component psychological treatment of irritable bowel syndrome. *Behaviour Research and Therapy*, 30 (2): 175–89.

Blanchard, E.B., Greene, B., Scharff, L. and Schwartz-McMorris, S.P. (1993). Relaxation training as a treatment for irritable bowel syndrome. *Biofeedback and Self Regulation*, 18 (3): 125–32.

Bridges, K.W. and Goldberg, D.P. (1985). Somatic presentation of DSM III psychiatric disorders in primary care. *Journal of Psychosomatic Research*, 29 (6): 563–9.

Bridges, K.W., Goldberg, D.P. and Evans, G.B. (1991). Determinants of somatisation in primary care. *Psychological Medicine*, 21: 473–83.

Burns, B.H. and Nichols, M.A. (1972). Factors related to the localisation of symptoms to the chest in depression. *British Journal of Psychiatry*, 121: 405–9.

Burns, D.D. (1980). *Feeling Good.* New York: New American Library.

Burns, D.D. and Nolen-Hoeksema, S. (1992). Therapeutic empathy and recovery from depression in cognitive behavioural therapy: a structural equation model. *Journal of Consulting and Clinical Psychology*, 60 (3): 441–9.

Cheyne, G. (1733). *The English Malady: or a Treatise of Nervous Diseases of all Kinds.* London: G. Strahan.

Clark, D.M. (1986). A cognitive approach to panic. *Behaviour Research and Therapy*, 24: 461–70.

Clark, D.M. (1989). Anxiety states. Panic and generalised anxiety. In K. Hawton, P.M. Salkovskis, J. Kirk and D.M. Clark (eds) *Cognitive Behaviour Therapy for Psychiatric Problems.* Oxford: Oxford University Press. pp. 52–96.

Craig, T.K.J. (1989). Abdominal pain. In G.W. Brown and T.O. Harris (eds). *Life Events and Illness.* New York: Guildford Press. pp. 233–59.

Craig, T.K.J. and Boardman, A.P. (1990). Somatisation in primary care settings. In C. Boss (ed.). *Somatisation: Physical Symptoms and Psychological Illness.* Oxford: Blackwell Scientific Publications. pp. 73–103.

Craig, T.K.J., Boardman, A.P., Mills, K., Daly-Jones, O. and Drake, H. (1993). The South London somatisation study. I: Longitudinal course and the influence of early life experiences. *British Journal of Psychiatry*, 163: 579–88.

Creed, F. (1995). Psychological treatment of the Irritable Bowel Syndrome and abdominal pain. In R. Mayou, C. Bass and M. Sharpe (eds). *Treatment of Functional Somatic Symptoms.* Oxford: Oxford University Press. pp. 255–70.

Creed, F. and Guthrie, E. (1993). Techniques for interviewing the somatising patient. *British Journal of Psychiatry*, 162: 467–71.

Creed, F., Mayou, R. and Hopkins, A. (eds) (1992). *Medical Symptoms not Explained by Organic Disease.* London: Royal College of Psychiatrists.

Day, R.W. and Sparacio, R.T. (1989). Structuring the counselling process. In W. Dryden (ed.). *Key Issues for Counselling in Action.* London: Sage. pp. 16–25.

DeRubeis, R.J. and Feeley, M. (1990). Determinants of change in cognitive therapy for depression. *Cognitive Therapy and Research*, 14 (5): 469–82.

Drossman, D.A., McKee, D.C., Sandler, R.S., Mitchell, C.M., Cramer, E.M., Lowman, B.C. and Burger, A.M. (1988). Psychosocial factors in the irritable bowel syndrome. A multivariate study of patients and non-patients with irritable bowel syndrome. *Gastroenterology*, 95: 701–8.

Drossman, D.A., Leserman, J., Nachman, G., Li, Z.M., Gluck, H., Toomey, T.C. and Mitchell, C.M. (1990). Sexual and physical abuse in women with functional or organic gastrointestinal disorders. *Annals of Internal Medicine*, 113: 828–33.

Dryden, W. (1989a). *Key Issues for Counselling in Action*. London: Sage.

Dryden, W. (1989b). The therapeutic alliance as an integrating framework. In W. Dryden (ed.). *Key Issues for Counselling in Action*. London: Sage. pp. 1–15.

Edwards, D.J.A. (1990). Cognitive therapy and the restructuring of early memories through guided imagery. *Journal of Cognitive Psychotherapy: An International Quarterly*, 4 (1): 33–50.

Ehlers, A. (1993). Somatic symptoms and panic attacks: A retrospective study of learning experiences. *Behaviour Research and Therapy*, 31 (3): 269–78.

Escobar, J.I., Burnam, A., Karno, M., Forsythe, A. and Golding, J.M. (1987). Somatisation in the community. Archives of *General Psychiatry*, 44: 713–18.

Farthing, M.J.G. (1995). Irritable bowel, irritable body or irritable brain? *British Medical Journal*, 310: 171–6.

Fennell, M.J.V. (1989). Depression. In K. Hawton, P.M. Salkovskis, J. Kirk and D.M. Clark (eds). *Cognitive Behaviour Therapy for Psychiatric Problems*. Oxford: Oxford University Press. pp. 169–234.

Fernandez, E. and Turk, D.C. (1989). The utility of cognitive coping strategies for altering pain perception: a meta-analysis. *Pain*, 38 (2): 123–36.

Freeman, A. (1992). The development of treatment conceptualizations in cognitive therapy. In A. Freeman and F.M. Dattilio (eds). *Comprehensive Casebook of Cognitive Therapy*. New York: Plenum Press. pp. 13–23.

Freeman, A., Pretzer, J., Fleming, B. and Simon, K. (1990). *Clinical Applications of Cognitive Therapy*. New York: Plenum Press.

Gask, L., Goldberg, D., Porter, R. and Creed, F. (1989). The treatment of somatisation: evaluation of a teaching package with general practice trainees. *Journal of Psychosomatic Research*, 33 (6): 697–703.

Gilbert, P. (1992). *Counselling for Depression*. London: Sage.

Goldberg, D.P. and Bridges, K.W. (1988). Somatic presentations of psychiatric illness in primary care settings. *Journal of Psychosomatic Research*, 32: 137–44.

Goldberg, D., Gask, L. and O'Dowd, T. (1989). The treatment of somatisation: teaching techniques of reattribution. *Journal of Psychosomatic Research*, 33 (6): 689–95.

Goldberg, R.J., Novack, D.H. and Gask, L. (1992). The recognition and management of somatisation. *Psychosomatics*, 33 (1): 55–61.

Greenberger, D. and Padesky, C. (1995). *Mind Over Mood*. New York: Guildford Press.

Griffith, J.L., Griffith, M.E. and Slovik, L.S. (1989). Mind-body patterns of symptom generation. *Family Process*, 28: 137–52.

Guthrie, E. (1995). Treatment of functional somatic symptoms: Psychodynamic Treatment. In R. Mayou, C. Bass and M. Sharpe (eds). *The Treatment of Functional Somatic Symptoms*. Oxford: Oxford University Press. pp. 144–60.

Guthrie, E., Creed, F., Dawson, D. and Tomenson, B. (1991). A controlled trial of psychological treatment for the irritable bowel syndrome. *Gastroenterology*, 100: 450–7.

Guthrie, E., Creed, F. and Whorwell, P.K. (1992). Outpatients with irritable bowel syndrome: a comparison of first time and chronic attenders. *Gut*, 33: 361–3.

Guthrie, E., Creed, F., Dawson, D. and Tomenson, B. (1993). A randomised controlled trial of psychotherapy in patients with refractory irritable bowel syndrome. *British Journal of Psychiatry*, 163: 315–21.

Hallam, R. (1992). *Counselling for Anxiety Problems*. London: Sage.

Hartvig, P. and Sterner, G. (1985). Childhood psychologic environmental exposure in women with diagnosed somatoform disorders. *Scandinavian Journal of Social Medicine*, 13: 153–7.

Harvey, R.F., Mauad, E.C. and Brown, A.M. (1987). Prognosis in the irritable bowel syndrome: a five year prospective study. *Lancet*, i: 963–5.

Hawton, K., Salkovskis, P.M., Kirk, J. and Clark, D.M. (eds) (1989). *Cognitive Behaviour Therapy for Psychiatric Problems*. Oxford: Oxford University Press.

Jacobson, N.S. (1989). The therapist-client relationship in cognitive behaviour therapy: implications for treating depression. *Journal of Cognitive Psychotherapy: An International Quarterly*, 3 (2): 85–96.

Katon, W., Von Korff, M., Lin, E., Lipscomb, P., Russon, J., Wagner, E. and Polk, E. (1990). Distressed high utilisers of medical care. DSM-III-R diagnoses and treatment needs. *General Hospital Psychiatry*, 12: 355–62.

Kellner, R., Hernandez, J. and Pathak, D. (1992). Self rated inhibited anger, somatisation and depression. *Psychotherapy and Psychosomatics*, 57: 102–7.

Kettell, J., Jones, R. and Lydeard, S. (1992). Reasons for consultation in irritable bowel syndrome: symptoms and patient characteristics. *British Journal of General Practice*, 42: 459–61.

Kiesler, D.J. (1988). *Therapeutic metacommunication: therapist impact disclosure as feedback in psychotherapy*. Palo Alto, CA: Consulting Psychologists Press.

Kirk, J. (1989). Cognitive behavioural assessment. In K. Hawton, P.M. Salkovskis, J. Kirk and D.M. Clark (eds). *Cognitive Behaviour Therapy for Psychiatric Problems*. Oxford: Oxford University Press. pp. 13–51.

Kirmayer, L.J. and Robbins, J.M. (eds) (1991). *Current Concepts of Somatisation. Research and Clinical Perspectives*. Washington DC: American Psychiatric Press.

Kleinman, A. and Kleinman, J. (1985). Somatisation: the interconnections in Chinese society among culture, depressive experiences and the meanings of pain. In A. Kleinman and B. Good (eds). *Culture and Depression*. California: University of California Press.

Klimes, I., Mayou, R.A., Pearce, M.J., Coles, L. and Fagg, J.R. (1990). Psychological treatment for atypical non-cardiac chest pain: a controlled evaluation. *Psychological Medicine*, 20: 605–11.

Kriechman, A.M. (1987). Siblings with somatoform disorders in childhood and adolescence. *Journal of the American Academy of Child and Adolescence Psychiatry*, 26: 226–31.

Lantinga, L.J., Sprafkin, R.P., McCroskery, J.H., Baker, M.T., Warner, R.A. and Hill, N.E. (1988). One year psychosocial follow-up of patients with chest pain and angiographically normal coronary arteries. *American Journal of Cardiology*, 62: 209–13.

Layden, M.A., Newman, C.F., Freeman, A. and Morse, S.B. (1993). *Cognitive Therapy of Borderline Personality Disorder*. Boston, MA: Allyn and Bacon.

Lipowski, Z.J. (1988). Somatisation: the concept and its clinical applications. *American Journal of Psychiatry*, 145: 1358–68.

Litt, M.D. and Baker, L.H. (1987). Cognitive behavioural intervention for irritable bowel syndrome. *Journal of Clinical Gastroenterology*, 9 (2): 208–11.

Lloyd, G.G. (1989). Somatisation: a psychiatrists perspective. *Journal of Psychosomatic Research*, 33 (6): 665–9.

Lydeard, S. and Jones, R. (1989). Factors affecting the decision to consult with dyspepsia: comparison of consulters and non-consulters. *British Journal of General Practice*, 39: 495–8.

Lynch, P.M. and Zamble, E. (1989). A controlled behavioural treatment study of irritable bowel syndrome. *Behaviour Therapy*, 20: 509–23.

Malan, M.A. and Kolko, D.J. (1982). Paradoxical intention in the treatment of obsessional flatulence ruminations. *Journal of Behaviour Therapy and Experimental Psychiatry*, 13 (2): 167–72.

Mandeville, B. (1711). *A Treatise of the Hypochondriack and Hysterick Passions*. London: Dryden Leach.

Manthei, R.J. and Matthews, D.A. (1989). Helping the reluctant client to engage in counselling. In W. Dryden (ed.). *Key Issues for Counselling in Action*. London: Sage.

Mayou, R. (1989). Atypical chest pain. *Journal of Psychosomatic Research*, 33 (4): 393–406.

Mayou, R. (1993). Somatisation. *Psychotherapy and Psychosomatics*, 59: 69–83.

Mayou, R., Bass, C. and Sharpe, M. (eds) (1995). *The Treatment of Functional Somatic Symptoms*. Oxford: Oxford University Press.

Mechanic, D. (1980). The experience and reporting of common physical complaints. *Journal of Health and Social Behaviour*, 21: 146–55.

Mechanic, D. (1986). The concept of illness behaviour: culture, situation and personal predisposition. *Psychological Medicine*, 16: 1–7.

Mearns, D. and Dryden, W. (eds) (1990). *Experiences of Counselling in Action*. London: Sage.

Melson, M.J., Clark, R.D., Rynearson, E.K., Snyder, A.L. and Dortzbach, J. (1982). Short term intensive group psychotherapy for patients with 'functional' complaints. *Psychosomatics*, 23: 689–95.

Melzack, R. and Wall, P.D. (1988). *The Challenge of Pain*. Second Edition. London: Penguin.

Murphy, M. (1989). Somatisation: embodying the problem. *British Medical Journal*, 298: 3331–2.

Murphy, M. (1993). Psychological management of somatisation disorder. In M. Hodes and S. Moorey (eds). *Psychological Treatment in Disease and Illness*. London: Gaskell. pp. 65–87.

Newman, C.F. (1994). Understanding client resistance: methods for enhancing motivation to change. *Cognitive and Behavioural Practice*, 1: 47–69.

Nielsen, G., Barth, K., Haver, B., Havik, O.E., Mølstad, E., Rogge, H. and Skåtun, M. (1988). Brief dynamic psychotherapy for patients presenting physical symptoms. *Psychotherapy and Psychosomatics*, 50: 35–41.

Padesky, C. (1993). Schema as self prejudice. *International Cognitive Therapy Newsletter*, 5/6: 16–17.

Padesky, C. and Mooney, K. (1990). Clinical tip. Presenting the cognitive model to clients. *International Cognitive Therapy Newsletter*, 6: 13–14.

Palmer, S. and Dryden, W. (1995). *Counselling for Stress Problems*. London: Sage.

Pearce, M.J., Mayou, R.A. and Klimes, I. (1990). The management of atypical non-cardiac chest pain. *Quarterly Journal of Medicine*, 281: 991–6.

Pennebaker, J.W. and Susman, J.R. (1988). Disclosure of traumas and psychosomatic processes. *Social Science and Medicine*, 26: 327–32.

Pennebaker, J.W. and Watson, D. (1991). The psychology of somatic symptoms. In L.J. Kirmayer and J.M. Robbins (eds). *Current Concepts of Somatisation. Research and Clinical Perspectives.* Washington DC: American Psychiatric Press.

Persons, J.B. (1989). *Cognitive Therapy in Practice. A Case Formulation Approach.* New York: W.W. Norton and Company.

Persons, J.B. (1993). Case conceptualization in cognitive behaviour therapy. In K.T. Kuehlwein and H. Rosen (eds). *Cognitive Therapies in Action. Evolving Innovative Practice.* San Francisco, CA: Jossey-Bass. pp. 33–53.

Persons, J.B. and Burns, D.D. (1985). Mechanisms of action in cognitive therapy: the relative contributions of technical and interpersonal interventions. *Cognitive Therapy and Research,* 9: 539–57.

Philips, H.C. (1987). The effect of behavioural treatment on chronic pain. *Behaviour Research and Therapy,* 25: 365–77.

Philips, H.C. (1988). *The Psychological Management of Chronic Pain: A Manual.* New York: Springer.

Porter, M. and Gorman, D. (1989). Approaches to somatisation. *British Medical Journal,* 298: 1332–3.

Potts, S.G. and Bass, C. (1994). Chest pain with normal coronary arteries: psychological aspects. In J.C. Kaski (ed.). *Angina Pectoris with Normal Coronary Arteries: Syndrome X.* Boston, MA: Kluwer.

Robbins, J.M. and Kirmayer, L.J. (1991). Cognitive and social factors in somatisation. In L.J. Kirmayer and J.M. Robbins (eds). *Current Concepts of Somatisation. Research and Clinical Perspectives.* Washington DC: American Psychiatric Press.

Rogers, C.R. (1957). The necessary and sufficient conditions of therapeutic personality change. *Journal of Consulting and Clinical Psychology,* 21: 95–103.

Roll, M. and Theorell, T. (1987). Acute chest pain without obvious organic cause before age 40 – personality and recent life events. *Journal of Psychosomatic Research,* 31: 215–21.

Safran, J.D. (1990). Towards a refinement of cognitive therapy in the light of interpersonal theory. Parts 1 and 2. *Clinical Psychology Review,* 10: 87–121.

Safran, J.D. and Segal Z.V. (1990). *Interpersonal Processes in Cognitive Therapy.* New York: Basic Books.

Salkovskis, P.M. (1989). Somatic problems. In K. Hawton, P.M. Salkovskis, J. Kirk and D.M. Clark (eds). *Cognitive Behaviour Therapy for Psychiatric Problems.* Oxford: Oxford University Press. pp. 235–76.

Salkovskis, P.M. (1991). The importance of behaviour in the maintenance of panic and anxiety: a cognitive account. *Behavioural Psychotherapy,* 19: 6–19.

Salkovskis, P.M. (1992a). The cognitive behavioural approach. In F. Creed, R. Mayou and A. Hopkins (eds). *Medical Symptoms not Explained by Organic Disease.* London: Royal College of Psychiatrists.

Salkovskis, P.M. (1992b). Psychological treatment of non cardiac chest pain: the cognitive approach. *American Journal of Medicine,* 92 (suppl. 5A): 114–21.

Salkovskis, P.M. and Warwick, H.M.C. (1986). Morbid preoccupations, health anxiety and reassurance: a cognitive-behavioural approach to hypochondriasis. *Behaviour Research and Therapy,* 24 (5): 597–602.

Sharpe, M. (1995). Cognitive behavioural therapies in the treatment of functional somatic syndromes. In R. Mayou, C. Bass and M. Sharpe (eds). *The Treatment of Functional Somatic Symptoms.* Oxford: Oxford University Press. pp. 122–43.

Sharpe, M., Peveler, R. and Mayou, R. (1992). The psychological treatment of patients with functional somatic symptoms. A practical guide. *Journal of Psychosomatic Research*, 36: 515–29.

Sharpe, M., Bass, C. and Mayou, R. (1995). An overview of the treatment of functional somatic symptoms. In R. Mayou, C. Bass and M. Sharpe (eds). *The Treatment of Functional Somatic Symptoms*. Oxford: Oxford University Press. pp. 66–86.

Sifneos, P.E. (1987). *Short term dynamic psychotherapy*. Second Edition. New York: Plenum Medical Books.

Skinner, J.B., Erskine, A., Pearce, S., Rubenstein, I., Taylor, M., Forster, C. (1990). The evaluation of a cognitive behavioural treatment programme in outpatients with chronic pain. *Journal of Psychosomatic Research*, 34: 13–19.

Spoto, G. and Williams, P. (1987). A 26 year old man with a fear of faecal incontinence. *Hospital Update*, September: 697–700.

Stern, R. and Fernandez, M. (1991). Group cognitive and behavioural treatment for hypochondriasis. *British Medical Journal*, 303: 1229–31.

Stevens, R. and Jones, R. (1993). Functional bowel disorders. In R. Jones (ed.). *Gastrointestinal Problems in General Practice*. Oxford: Oxford University Press. pp. 126–35.

Sulloway, F. (1979). *Freud: Biologist of the Mind*. New York: Basic Books.

Surawy, C., Hackmann, A., Hawton, K. and Sharpe, M. (1995). Chronic fatigue syndrome: a cognitive approach. *Behaviour Research and Therapy*, 33 (5): 535–44.

Svedlund, J., Sjodin, I., Ottosson, J. and Dotevall, G. (1983). Controlled study of psychotherapy in irritable bowel syndrome. *Lancet*, ii: 589–92.

Swarbrick, E.T., Hegarty, J.E., Bat, L., Williams, C.B. and Dawson, A.M. (1980). Site of pain from the irritable bowel. *Lancet*, ii: 443–6.

Taylor, G.J. (1987). *Psychosomatic Medicine and Contemporary Psychoanalysis*. International Universities Press, Stress and Health Series, Monograph Number 3. Madison, CT: International Universities Press.

Thompson, W.G., Creed, F., Drossman, D.A., Heaton, K.W. and Mazzacca, G. (1992). Functional bowel disease and functional abdominal pain. *Gastroenterology International*, 5 (2): 75–91.

Toner, B.B. (1994). Cognitive behavioural treatment of functional somatic syndromes: integrating gender issues. *Cognitive and Behavioural Practice*, 1: 157–78.

Toner, B.B., Garfinkel, P.E. and Jeejeebhoy, K.N. (1990a). Psychological factors in irritable bowel syndrome. *Canadian Journal of Psychiatry*, 35 (2): 158–61.

Toner, B.B., Garfinkel, P.E., Jeejeebhoy, K.N., Scher, H., Shulhan, D. and Di-Gasbarro, I. (1990b). Self-schema in irritable bowel syndrome and depression. *Psychosomatic Medicine*, 52 (2): 149–55.

Toner, B.B., Koyama, E., Garfinkel, P.E., Jeejeebhoy, K.N. and Di-Gasbarro, I. (1992). Social desirability and irritable bowel syndrome. *International Journal of Psychiatry in Medicine*, 22 (1): 99–103.

Trower, P., Casey, A. and Dryden, W. (1988). *Cognitive Behavioural Counselling in Action*. London: Sage.

Walker, E.A., Katon, W.J., Harrop-Griffiths, J., Holm, L., Russo, J. and Hickok, L.R. (1988). Relationship of chronic pelvic pain to psychiatric diagnoses and childhood sexual abuse. *American Journal of Psychiatry*, 145: 75–80.

Walker, E.A., Katon, W.J., Hansom, J., Harrop-Griffiths, J., Holm, L., Jones, M.L., Hickok, L.R. and Jemelka, P. (1992). Medical and psychiatric symptoms in women with childhood sexual abuse. *Psychosomatic Medicine*, 54: 658–64.

Walker, E.A., Katon, W.J., Roy-Byrner, P.P., Jemelka, R.P. and Russo, J. (1993).

Histories of sexual victimisation in patients with irritable bowel syndrome or inflammatory bowel disease. *American Journal of Psychiatry*, 150 (10): 1502–6.

Ward, D.E. (1989). Termination of individual counselling: concepts and strategies. In W. Dryden (ed.). *Key Issues for Counselling in Action*. London: Sage. pp. 97–110.

Warwick, H.M.C. (1989). A cognitive behavioural approach to hypochondriasis and health anxiety. *Journal of Psychosomatic Research*, 33 (6): 705–11.

Warwick, H.M.C. (1995). Treatment of hypochondriasis. In R. Mayou, C. Bass and M. Sharpe (eds). *The Treatment of Functional Somatic Symptoms*. Oxford: Oxford University Press. pp. 163–74.

Warwick, H.M.C. and Marks, I.M. (1988). Behavioural treatment of illness phobia and hypochondriasis. *British Journal of Psychiatry*, 152: 239–41.

Warwick, H.M.C. and Salkovskis, P.M. (1985). Reassurance. *British Medical Journal*, 290: 1028.

Warwick, H.M.C. and Salkovskis, P.M. (1989). Hypochondriasis. In J. Scott, J.M.C. Williams and A.T. Beck (eds). *Cognitive Therapy in Clinical Practice*. London: Croom Helm. pp. 78–102.

Warwick, H.M.C. and Salkovskis, P.M. (1990). Hypochondriasis. *Behaviour Research and Therapy*, 28 (2): 105–17.

Watson, J.P. (1985). Frame of reference and the detection of individual and systemic problems. *Journal of Psychosomatic Research*, 29: 571–7.

Wells, A. and Hackmann, A. (1993). Imagery and core beliefs in health anxiety: content and origins. *Behavioural and Cognitive Psychotherapy*, 21 (3): 265–74.

Whale, J. (1992). The use of brief focal psychotherapy in the treatment of chronic pain. *Psychoanalytic Psychotherapy*, 6 (1): 61–72.

Whorwell, P.J., Prior, A. and Faragher, B. (1984). Controlled trial of hypnotherapy in the treatment of severe refractory irritable bowel syndrome. *Lancet*, ii: 1232–4.

Wilkinson, P. and Mynors-Wallis, L. (1994). Problem solving therapy in the treatment of unexplained physical symptoms in primary care: A preliminary study. *Journal of Psychosomatic Research*, 38 (6): 591–8.

World Health Organization (1993). *The ICD-10 Classification of Mental and Behavioural Disorders*. Geneva: World Health Organization.

Wright, J.H. and Davis, D. (1994). The therapeutic relationship in cognitive behavioural therapy: patient perceptions and therapist responses. *Cognitive and Behavioural Practice*, 1: 25–45.

Yalom, I.D. (1975). *The Theory and Practice of Group Psychotherapy* Second Edition. New York: Basic Books.

Young, J.E. (1990). *Cognitive Therapy for Personality Disorders: A Schema Focused Approach*. Sarasota, FL: Personal Resource Exchange.

Young, J.E. and Klosko, J.S. (1993). *Reinventing Your Life*. London: Penguin.

Index

ABC technique 84–5
abuse 30–1, 110–11; and bowel disorders 31; and hypochondriasis 31; and pelvic pain 31
activity: increasing 87–8; and pain 88
agenda setting 55–6, 77–8
alexythymia 3, 29
alternative medicine: *see* complementary medicine
anger: towards medical profession 121–2
angina: and atypical chest pain 4, 5, 23, 25, 44, 45, 69, 96
anxiety: and physical symptoms 5–7, 16–17; about health 1, 6, 11, 18, 35
assessment 53–74; agenda for 55–6; aims 56–7; and avoidance 66; and coping strategies 64–6; and development of problems 67–8; and family history 68–9; and health beliefs 66–7; and interpersonal factors 70–1; and life events 70; and maintenance of problems 59–66; and mood 69–70; skills 58–9; stages 59–71; and stress 70; and triggers 64
assumptions 15, 26–35, 66–7; 99–109; 110–11; characteristics 100–1; counsellors' 48; identifying 99–101, 103–6; modifying 106–9, 110–11; skills in working with 102–3; *see also* beliefs
atypical chest pain 4, 8, 10, 23–6; and angina 4, 5, 23, 25, 44, 45, 69, 96; case study 60–1, 80–1, 82–3, 92, 106, 108, 111, 132–3; causes 23; cognitive model 23–6; definition 23; and effectiveness of counselling 36; frequency 10, 23; and heart disease 23, 44–5; and hyperventilation 25, 82; and life events 24; and psychological problems 23; and safety behaviours 25; and stress 24

avoidance 35, 66; assessment of 66; modifying 87–8; *see also* safety behaviours

back pain 7
Barsky, A.J. 31
Beck, A.T. 14, 26
behaviour therapy 14, 35
behavioural experiments: *see* experiments
belief ratings 66–7, 86
beliefs 15, 26–35, 99–111; characteristics 100–1; counsellors 48; definition 26, 99–101; health 8, 10, 66–7; identifying 103–6; modifying 109–11; about psychological distress 29–34; about self 28; skills in working with 102–3; *see also* assumptions, schema
bereavement 11–12; *see also* grief
blueprint 132
body dysmorphic disorder 9
body sensations 15–16
bowel problems: *see* irritable bowel syndrome
breathing control 90; *see also* hyperventilation
breathlessness 4, 6, 17, 89; and hyperventilation 82
Breuer, J. 3
Bridges, K.W. 7
broadening the agenda 41–2
Briquet's syndrome 9; *see also* multiple symptoms, somatization disorder

case conceptualization: *see* conceptualization
case study: atypical chest pain 60–1, 80–1, 82–3, 92, 106, 108, 111, 132–3; irritable bowel syndrome 61–5, 67–8, 73, 91–2, 94, 104, 105, 107–8, 129–30
chest pain: *see* atypical chest pain